Key Concepts

STEM

SCIENCE TECHNOLOGY ENGINEERING MATH

ENGINEERING AND TECHNOLOGY

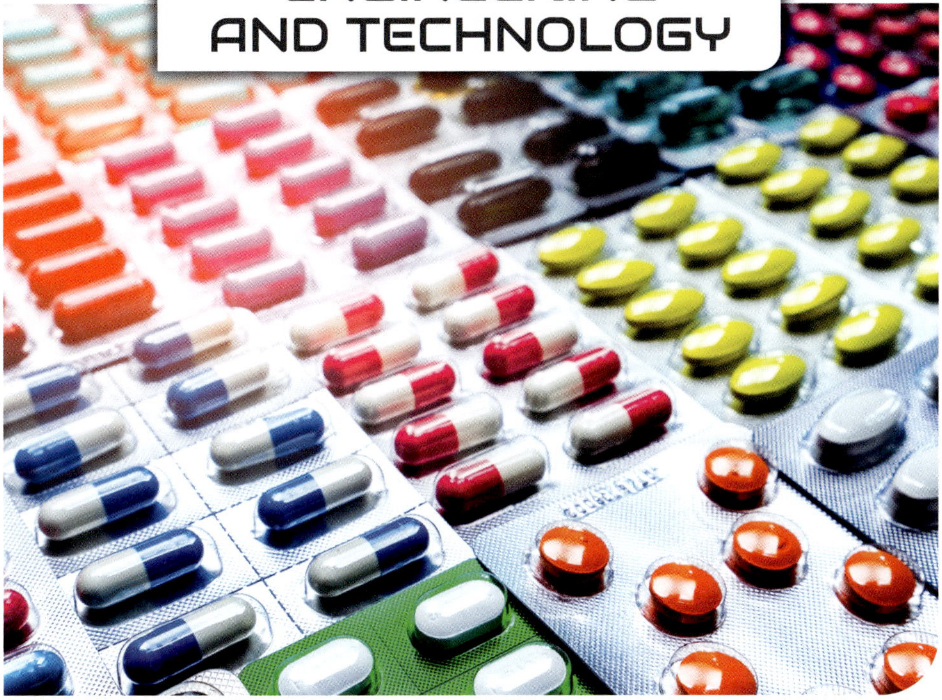

MEDICINE AND HEALTH

General Editor: Anne O'Daly

BROWN BEAR BOOKS

Published by Brown Bear Books Ltd
4877 N. Circulo Bujia, Tucson, AZ 85718
USA
and
Studio G14, Regent Studios, 1 Thane Villas,
London N7 7PH, UK

Cataloging-in-Publication data available upon request.

ISBN 978-1-83572-063-9 (ALB)
ISBN 978-1-83572-069-1 (paperback)
ISBN 978-1-83572-075-2 (ebook)

Children's Publisher: Anne O'Daly
Design Manager: Keith Davis
Picture Manager: Sophie Mortimer
Consultant: Chris Woodford

Manufactured in the United States of America
CPSIA compliance information: Batch#AG/5664

Picture Credits
Front Cover: Shutterstock: Bk87. **Interior: iStock:** Kali9 59, wynnter 8b, Matthew Wzinder 14, 26bl; **Library of Congress:** 22b; **Photos.com:** 4–5, 7t, 10, 16t, 17, 18br, 19, 20t, 36t, 41b; Public Domain: Alokprasad 41t, Cantonal Museum of Archeology and History 5, lensonleeuwenhoek.net 16br, Manske, Magnus/digital collections/hst/scientific 11t, NLM 8t, Popular historia 18bl, 60, Yassine M Rabet 16bl; **Shutterstock:** Ammu67 26br, antb 7b, Juan Miguel Aparicio 51, Appalachian trail 34b, Ann Areeya 25, ChameleionsEye 55, daphnusia 49t, Dragon Images 33b, Fahroni 1, 22t, Ekaterina Georgivskia 56t, gopixa 58t, Gorodenkoff 12-13t, 49b, Doro Guzenda 35r, Rohane Hamilton 56b, Lis Kiryl 42t, Denis Kornilv 4bl, Dmitri Ma 27t, Maksimilian 28, Kallayanee Naloka 26cr, Mis Natali 30t, chakkrachai nicharat 23t, Hein Nouwens 36b, Tyler Olson 29, Andrey Popov 34t, Aexander Raths 32, SpringSky 39, Stock 52t, triocean 33t, UfaBizPhoto 40, 61, uno1 30b, Martin Valigursky 52b, Fam Veld 50, Roman Zaiets 48; **Thinkstock:** Hemera 6t, PhotoObjecs.net 35l; **Topfoto:** World History Archive 15, 23b; **United States Government:** Department of Health and Human Services/Centers for Disease Control and Prevention 20b; **Wellcome Images:** 6b, 13.

Brown Bear Books has made every attempt to contact the copyright holder. If you have any information about omissions please contact licensing@brownbearbooks.co.uk.

STEM

Key Concepts in STEM: Engineering and Technology describes the scientific principles and feats of engineering that have shaped the world we live in. Since earliest times, people have created tools and machines to provide shelter, warmth, security, and protection from disease. This book describes the advances that have taken place in medicine and healthcare since earliest times. In the last 100 years, discoveries and technical innovations have meant that many ensured that many conditions that were once fatal can now be treated. The book also looks at advances in gene therapy and the uses of artificial intelligence in medical care. Explanatory diagrams and informative photographs explain how STEM (science, technology, engineering, and math) has transformed our lives and continues to influence our world today.

Publisher's note to educators and parents: Our editors have carefully reviewed the web sites included at the end of this book to ensure that they are suitable for students. Many web sites change frequently, however, and we cannot guarantee that a site's future contents will continue to meet our high standards of quality and educational value. Be advised that students should be closely supervised whenever they access the Internet.

Contents

EARLY MEDICINE

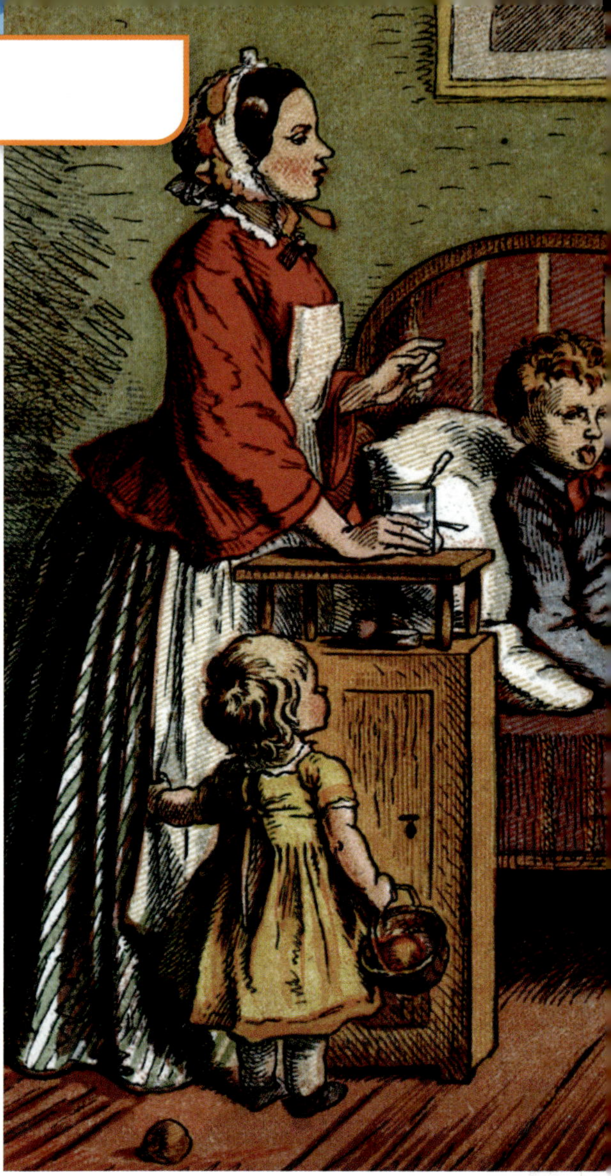

Modern medicine is a well-developed, sophisticated area of science, using advanced technology. But its more humble beginnings can be traced back thousands of years to prehistoric society.

Most prehistoric peoples lived in small groups and wandered from place to place, using materials such as bone, wood, and stone to construct simple tools. The study of their skeletons reveals that they could reset broken bones and perform minor operations, but they probably often believed that a sufferer from disease was possessed by an evil spirit.

SUPERNATURAL CURES

It was not only prehistoric peoples who thought diseases could be caused by magic and spirits. The ancient Egyptians, whose civilization began around 3000 BCE, were also firm believers in the supernatural. They often wore charms to keep evil spirits away, and if they did become ill, they usually turned to magic and their gods to cure them. The ancient Greeks and Romans constructed temples to Asclepius, the god of healing, to which sick people were often taken to receive miracle cures. Throughout the Middle Ages, when Christianity had become the main religion in Europe, sick people often went on pilgrimages to holy sites, hoping for relief. Even today, witch doctors who practice herbal medicine are important in parts of the world.

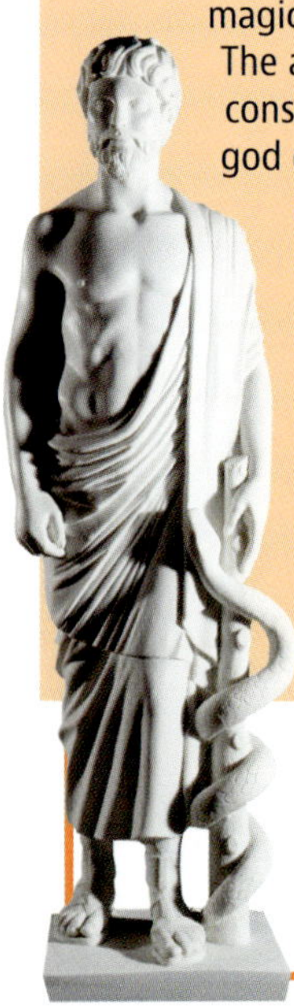

Asclepius, the Greek god of healing, carried a staff entwined with a snake. This symbol is still used by medical institutions.

One major operation performed by prehistoric people was trepanning, or cutting a hole in the skull of a person while they were still alive. Ancient trepanned skulls have been found in every part of the world. Many of the skulls have new bone growth around the edges of the hole, showing that the person probably lived on for many years after the operation.

Herbal Remedies

Ancient cures were often a combination of herbal and magical elements. Chest conditions

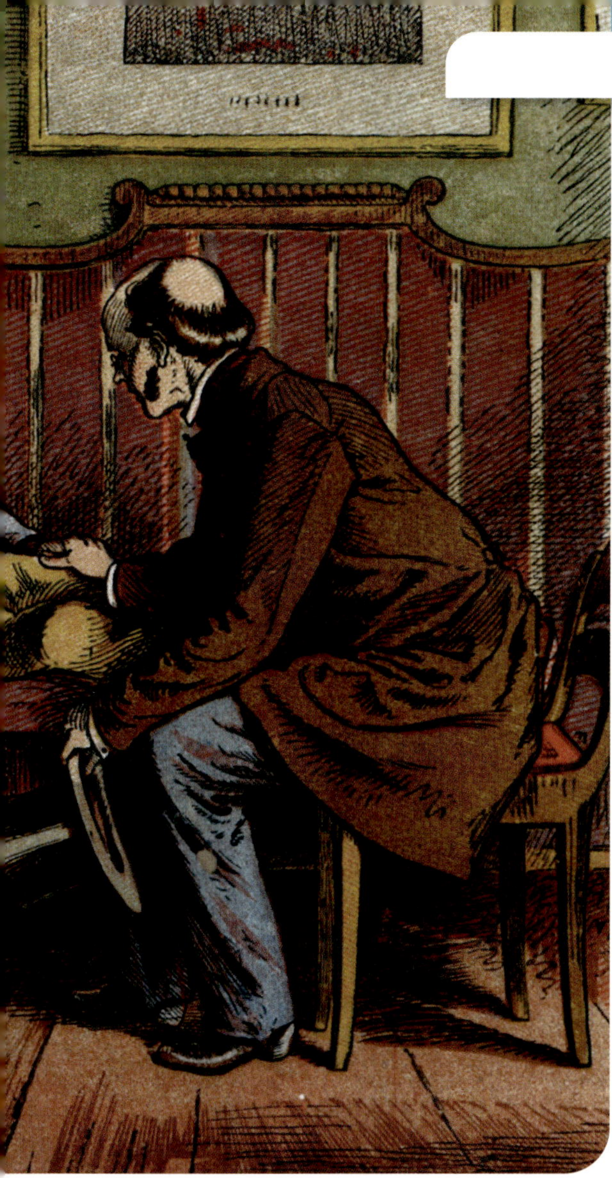

All illness was potentially deadly before medicines were invented, but calling for a doctor was expensive and so was often a last resort, even for wealthy families.

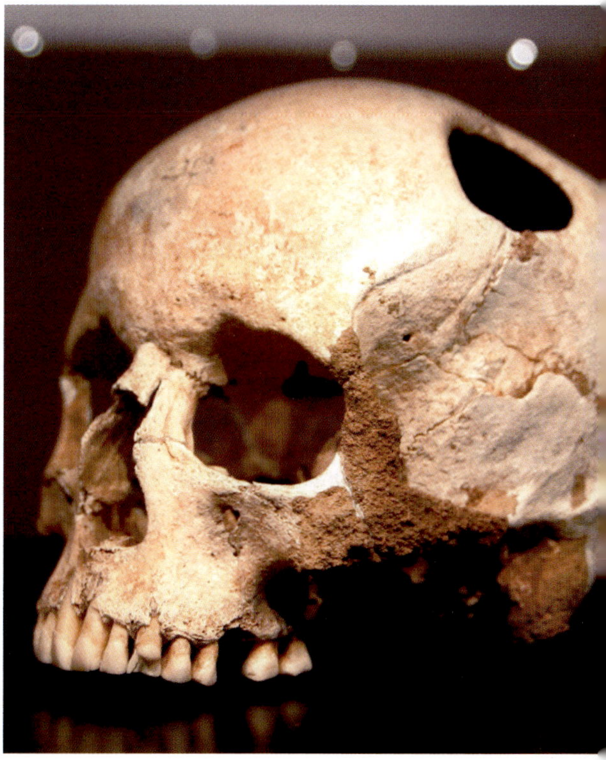

A prehistoric human skull with a hole in it from a trepanning procedure. These operations might have been carried out to relieve headaches or to release evil spirits.

were treated by making the patient inhale steam, while cuts and burns were treated with ointments. Often the doctor would chant spells or perform ceremonies as the treatment was administered. Egyptian records show that if a treatment worked, people continued to use it. Those treatments that failed were soon forgotten. In this way, the ancient Egyptians built up medical knowledge, and many of

BOOKS OF THOTH

The most important early Egyptian medical books were the *Books of Thoth*, kept by priests at the temple to Thoth, the Egyptian god of wisdom. Although none of these works has survived, researchers have found a medical book from around 1500 BCE, which was probably based on them. It contains detailed instructions on how to deal with many common illnesses.

their treatments are still used in some parts of the world. From the periods of Greek and Roman civilization to the end of the 18th century, herbal cures were widely used. New herbal treatments were always being added to the growing body of medical knowledge. However, there was little science involved in this area of medicine, and no one knew why the treatments worked. For example, it has been known for hundreds of years that the bark of willow trees and plants such as meadowsweet cures headaches when it is chewed. It was only in the 19th century that the substance responsible for this effect, salicylic acid, which is now used to make aspirin, was finally identified. Another century passed before it was understood how the substance worked on the human body. Although there are people who still rely on herbal remedies, scientific evidence for their effectiveness is limited in many cases.

The ancient Egyptians were the first to devise a theory of disease. This allowed them to develop treatments for serious illnesses in a systematic manner. Influenced by the seasonal rise and fall of the Nile River, which was important for Egyptian agriculture, doctors theorized that the human body must be full of channels for blood and other fluids. The blockage of one of these channels would lead to illness, and treatments such as emetics (substances that cause vomiting), laxatives, and bleeding (drawing out blood) were used to try and clear blockages and cure the patient.

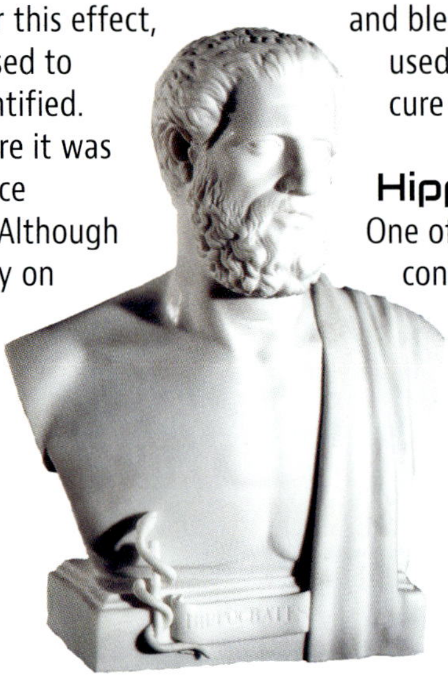

Hippocrates, the founder of modern medicine, rejected the idea that diseases had any kind of supernatural cause or that magic could be used as an important part of treatment.

Hippocrates

One of the greatest individual contributors to medical knowledge was a Greek physician called Hippocrates, who lived from around 460 BCE to 377 BCE. Very little is known about

CLINICAL OBSERVATION AND DIAGNOSIS

Hippocrates set out the principles of diagnosis. He observed symptoms to predict the course of the disease. Once a prognosis (prediction) had been made, he gave treatment while monitoring the patient. Modern doctors still use this approach today.

Later, doctors invented tests that made the diagnosis more precise. Temperature can be used to gauge sickness, for example. In 1626, an Italian physician called Santorio (1561–1636) invented a water thermometer that allowed doctors to measure temperature with greater accuracy. Medieval doctors listened to a patient's lungs and heart. A technique called percussion was developed by Austrian Leopold Auenbrügger (1722–1809). He tapped not only a patient's chest but also the abdomen to "listen in" to internal organs.

The microscope was first used to study disease by Athanasius Kircher (1602–1680). In 1646, he looked at the blood of plague victims, and believed he could see "little worms" that could be the cause of the disease.

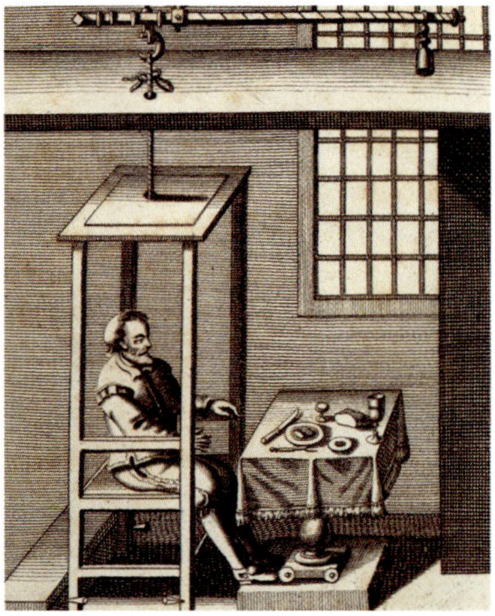

Santorio also invented a weighing machine for checking a person's own health.

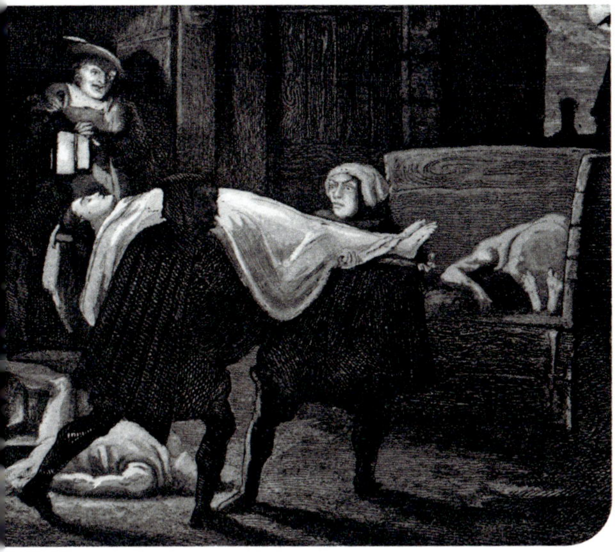

During Europe's Black Death epidemics, plague victims were collected from houses each night for immediate burial to try and prevent the still mysterious disease from spreading.

Hippocrates himself, but he is associated with a collection of medical texts that were written in around 430 BCE. Hippocrates devised his own theory of disease. He thought that the body was made up from four "humors"—blood, phlegm, black bile, and yellow bile. He suggested that in a healthy body the humors are all finely balanced, but if this balance is disrupted, illness results. His theory of disease was widely used by European doctors throughout the Middle Ages.

Anatomy

The ancient Egyptians made several advances in anatomy—the study of the structure of the body. They also learned how to preserve, or mummify, dead bodies, which they believed were still needed in the afterlife. Galen, a physician working in Rome in the 2nd century CE, dissected humans to study anatomy. Although many of his findings were incorrect, Galen's picture of the human body remained unchallenged for centuries.

HEALTH AND LIFESTYLE

The connection between cleanliness and health was probably first made by the ancient Egyptians, who washed their clothes and bodies regularly. Toilets and baths were common among the rich, and some Egyptians even slept under mosquito nets. Like the Egyptians, the Greeks and Romans also knew of the benefits of a healthy lifestyle. Greek physician Diocles, who lived in the 4th century BCE, advocated washing with pure water every day and even cleaning the teeth with peppermint-flavored powder. The Romans turned bathing into a social event, building great public baths in many of their cities.

With the fall of the Roman Empire in 476 CE, sewers and aqueducts (channels that carried fresh water into towns and cities) fell into disrepair, and living standards declined. Filthy streets and poor food and water hygiene contributed to outbreaks of infectious diseases during the Middle Ages. Conditions didn't begin to improve until the Industrial Revolution during the 19th century.

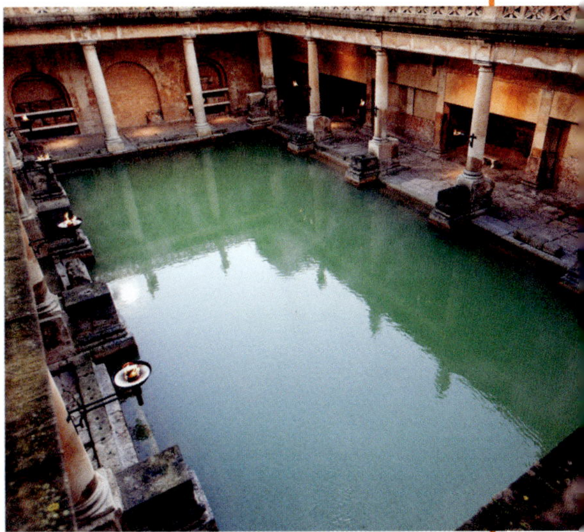

A public bath was a central part of a Roman city. Bathers plunged into pools of different temperatures, and used olive oil to clean the skin. Soap had not yet been invented.

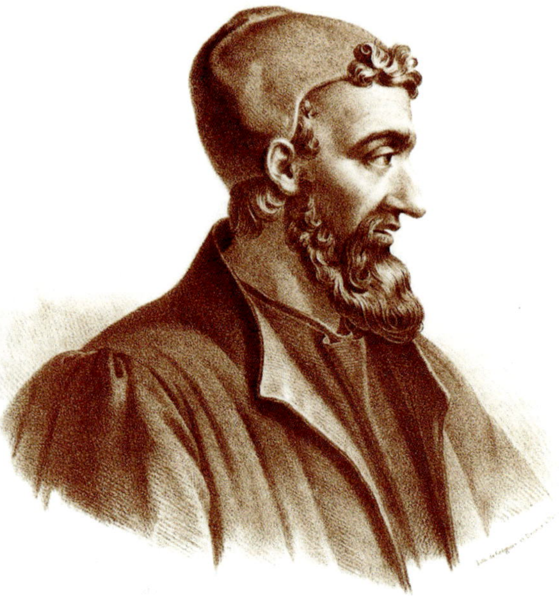

Galen was a doctor who practised in the Roman world in the 2nd century CE*.. His work influenced doctors until the 17th century.*

Gradually, knowledge of the workings of the human body improved during the early-modern period. Flemish anatomist Andreas Vesalius (1514–1564) was the first person to improve on Galen's theory of anatomy.

Blood Circulation

Vesalius drew detailed pictures of body systems, building up layer upon layer of anatomical features in the body. Vesalius's book *On the Fabric of the Human Body* (1543) corrected several of Galen's mistakes, but did not challenge Galen's view of blood movement. In 1559, Italian anatomist Realdo Colombo (1516–1559) showed that blood passed from one side of the heart to the other via the lungs. This finding led English physician and anatomist William Harvey (1578–1657) to demonstrate how blood circulated through the body. Tiny blood vessels, called capillaries, that ran through all body parts were discovered later by Italian anatomist Marcello Malpighi (1628–1694).

SOCIETY AND INVENTIONS

Hospitals and Medical Schools

The Romans needed healthy soldiers to sustain their empire and developed the first system of public health. State doctors were appointed to tend to the poor, and hospitals were built in many cities. Following the collapse of the western Roman world in the 5th century CE, however, doctors were in short supply. Poor people had to use herbal remedies. Barbers set bones, pulled teeth (*right*), and stitched wounds. The first medical school was set up around 1100 CE at Salerno in Italy. Soon similar schools were established all over Europe, but doctors and hospitals were still too expensive for most people and were only located in major cities. Widespread, affordable health care was not available until the 20th century.

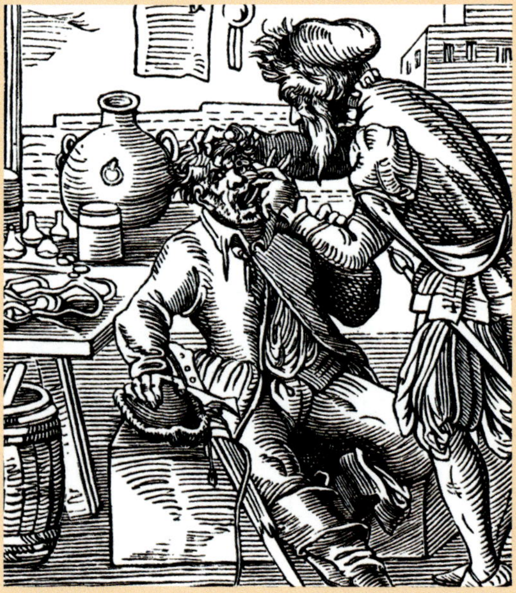

CIRCULATION OF THE BLOOD

The circulation of blood in the lungs was first described by Ibn al-Nafīs an Egyptian who lived in the 13th century.

William Harvey discovered how blood moved around the body in the early 17th century. His findings contradicted the theory proposed by Galen that had been taught for centuries. Galen thought that blood was made inside the heart and liver and drawn into the body where it was used up to be replaced by new blood. Harvey showed that if this were true, a body would be making 550 lb (250 kg) of blood per day.

Harvey saw that the heart was a four-chambered pump. As blood passes through the body, the oxygen that it carries is used up. This blood, called deoxygenated blood (shown in blue, *right*), then enters the right atrium (chamber) of the heart. From there it is pumped into the right ventricle and then to the lungs, where it absorbs more oxygen. Oxygen-carrying blood (red) passes back to the heart, entering the left atrium and flowing into the left ventricle, the most powerful chamber, which pumps the blood back to the tissues of the body.

Vessels that carry blood toward the heart are called veins, while those that carry blood away from the heart are arteries. Valves inside the veins and the heart stop blood flowing in the wrong direction.

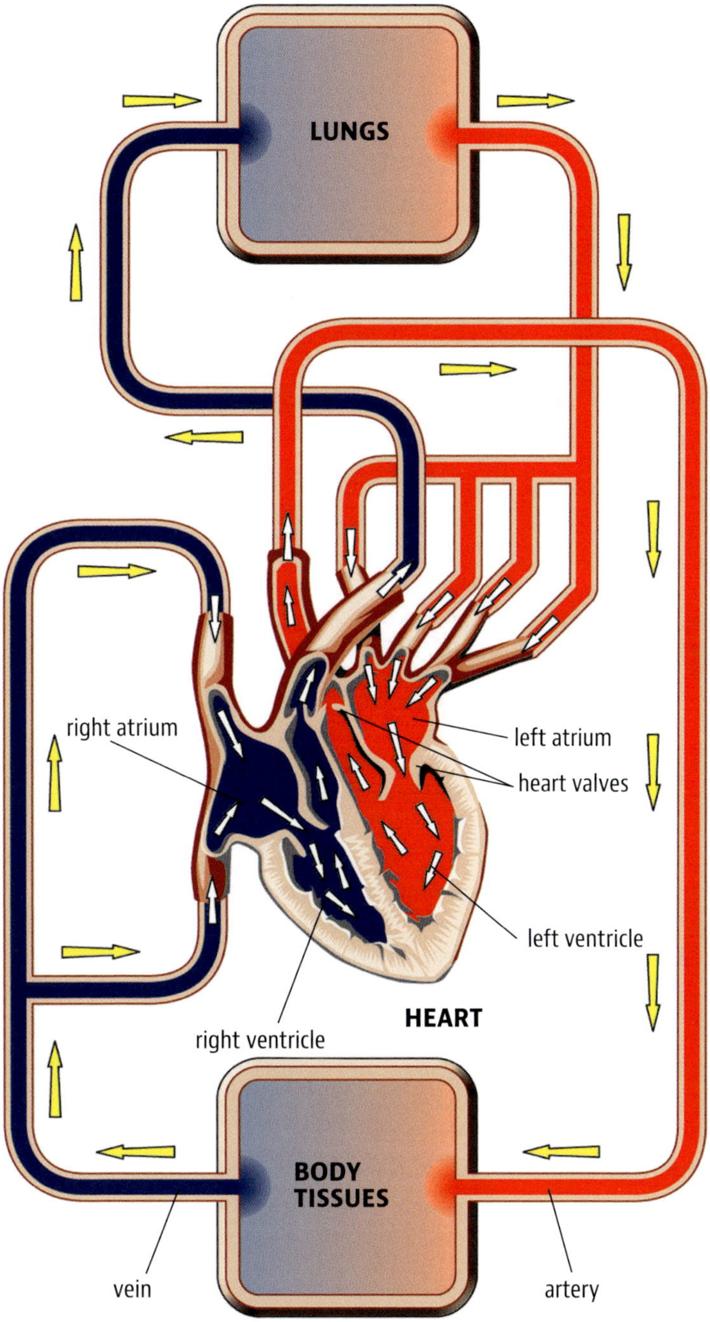

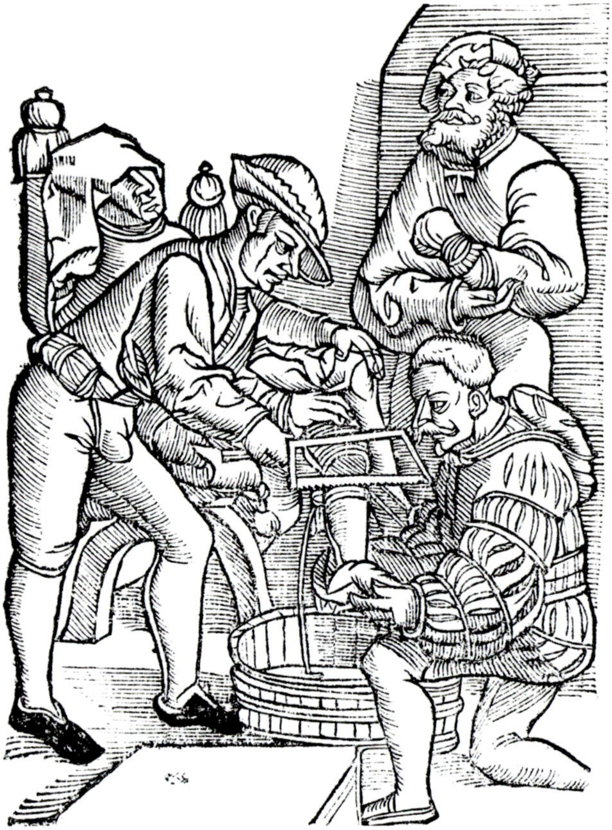

Early surgery, such as a leg amputation, was fast and brutal. The procedure happened while the patient was still awake.

SCIENCE WORDS

Plague: This term can refer to any epidemic (a widespread outbreak of disease) that claims many lives. A major outbreak of plague occurred in Europe around 542 CE. Another outbreak, between 1346 and 1353, claimed 25 million lives—almost a quarter of the total European population. Medieval doctors had no way of treating plague, and many lost their own lives to the disease.

Leprosy: One of the oldest known diseases (an Egyptian skeleton from around 500 BCE shows signs of it). With no effective treatments available, millions of people died from leprosy during the Middle Ages. Today the disease is still present in many parts of the world, and it is estimated that 10 million people suffer from it.

Syphilis: This disease had been identified in 4,000-year-old skeletons from central Russia, but the first European outbreak occurred in 1493. Sailors on Christopher Columbus's voyage may have carried the disease to Europe from the Americas. Early treatments involving herbal remedies and mercury proved ineffective. The disease incubated for many years in the body before entering a fatal final phase.

Surgery

Egyptian surgeons probably performed minor operations, such as the removal of cysts and lumps. Most were successful because wounds were treated with the leaves and bark of willow, which contains a natural antiseptic to kill germs. Surgery was hazardous in ancient Greece because human dissection was banned, and surgeons had very little knowledge of human anatomy. The work of Galen led to improvements, but much of this knowledge was lost with the fall of the Roman Empire around 476 CE.

Surgery was considered manual work in medieval Europe, and most doctors refused to perform it. Instead, operations were left to barbers, who mostly cut hair. The two main problems with surgery are pain and infection: medieval surgeons tried to tackle both. Italian surgeon Hugh of Lucca bathed wounds in wine to prevent infection, but the idea was not generally adopted. Attempts were made to dull pain by drugging patients or giving them large quantities of alcohol before operations, but these substances were not as effective as modern anaesthetics.

Ambroise Paré (1510–1590), a French surgeon, wrote several books that improved the standard of medieval surgery. He stressed the importance of avoiding excessive pain, advocating quick and simple operations, and condemning the use of cruel techniques such as cauterizing wounds (burning them) to stop bleeding.

Despite these advances, surgery continued to be dangerous until further advances in medicine became more scientifically based during the 19th century, around the time of the Industrial Revolution.

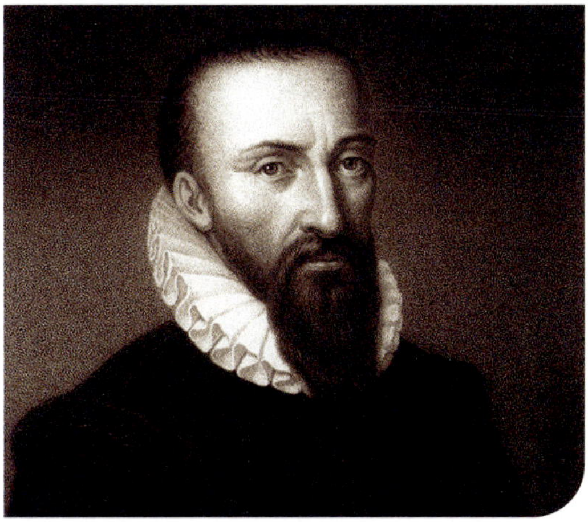

Ambroise Paré was a 16th-century French surgeon. He rediscovered a Roman ointment made from egg white and turpentine that stopped incisions from becoming infected.

ANCIENT EGYPTIAN SURGEON'S BAG

This relief is carved into the wall of an Egyptian temple at Kom Ombo that was built between 332 BCE and 395 CE. The relief is close to others showing medical scenes, such as the queen giving birth. Some scholars believe this relief (right) shows a selection of surgical tools. There are no written descriptions of the instruments, and the uses of all are not known, but tools that have been identified are listed below:

1 Knives probably used to make incisions (cuts) during operations.
2 A drill for making holes in bones or teeth.
3 A saw for cutting through bones.
4 Forceps and pincers to remove embedded objects such as thorns.
5 A censer, an object used in herbal medicine to burn incense.
6 Herbal cures inside cloth bags.
7 Magical charms in the shape of the eye of the Egyptian god Horus.
8 Scales for weighing herbal cures.
9 Cups for extracting blood.
10 A papyrus scroll.
11 Shears for cutting hair.
12 A sponge for cleaning wounds.
13 Spoons for administering cures.

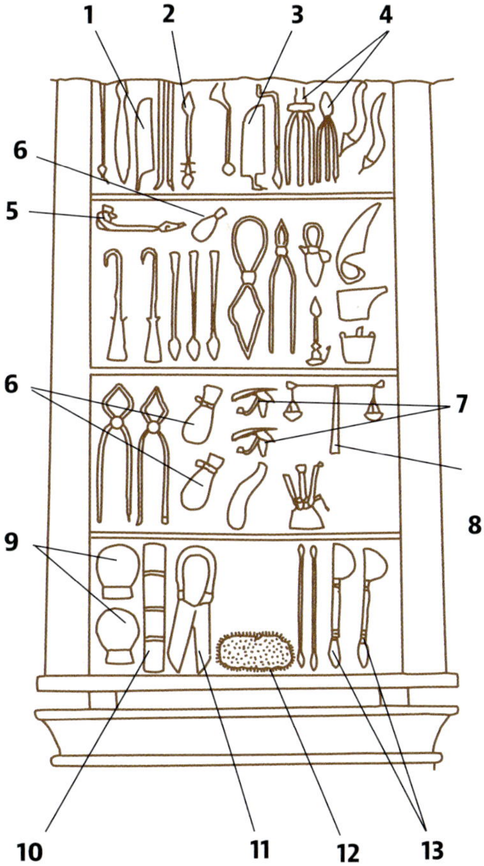

MEDICINE MEETS SCIENCE

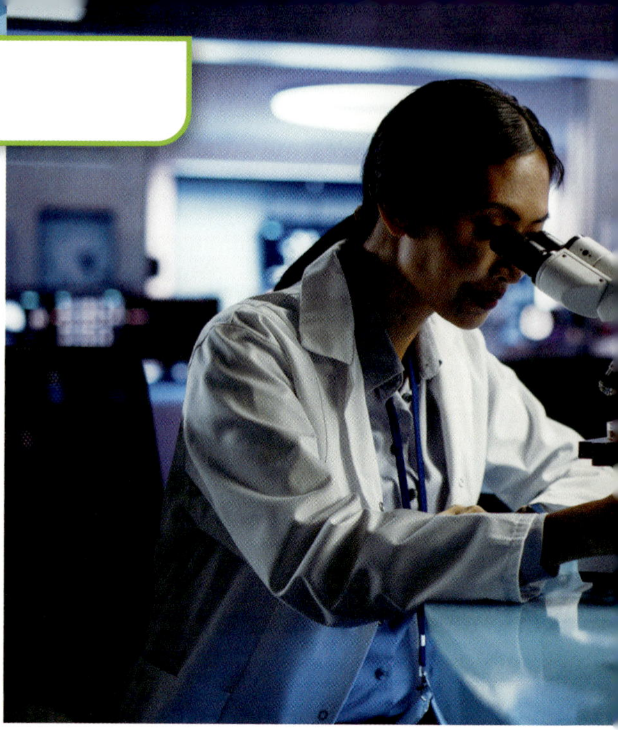

Medicine became more scientifically based in the 19th century. As a result, pain, infection, and many deadly diseases were overcome.

At the beginning of the 19th century, medicine had not really changed since the time of the ancient Greeks. Doctors thought that bad air, the climate, or a poor diet caused diseases. They did not realize the need for cleanliness to prevent infections. Hospitals were often filthy, and patients who went in for treatment had a high risk of becoming infected and dying as a result of their stay.

The most feared medical procedure was amputation—the surgical removal of a limb. At that time there was no effective pain relief for operations, and patients were usually tied down to the operating table after being forced to drink massive amounts of alcohol to numb the pain. However, during the century, medical treatment became safer due to the work of scientists who developed safe anesthetics (substances that relieve pain) and realized the importance of keeping hospitals and medical equipment free from microscopic germs such as bacteria and viruses.

Pain Relief

In 1848, a patient who had suffered an amputation said that someone preparing to undergo an operation was like "a condemned criminal preparing for an execution."

HYPODERMIC SYRINGE

Before the 19th century, most medicine was administered by mouth. Then, around 1850, French surgeon Charles Gabriel Pravaz (1791–1853) and Scottish doctor Alexander Wood (1817–1884) independently began injecting morphine beneath the skin using a syringe, a glass tube, and a plunger with a hollow metal needle. Pravaz and Wood found that this new method enabled them to control doses much more accurately. The drug also acted much faster and could be injected at the site where pain was worse. Before long, news of the invention traveled and use of hypodermic (the word means "under the skin") syringes became widespread. Today, glass tubes have been replaced with plastic ones. They have a scale marked so drug doses can be measured accurately. Modern syringe needles are disposed of rather than sterilized and reused.

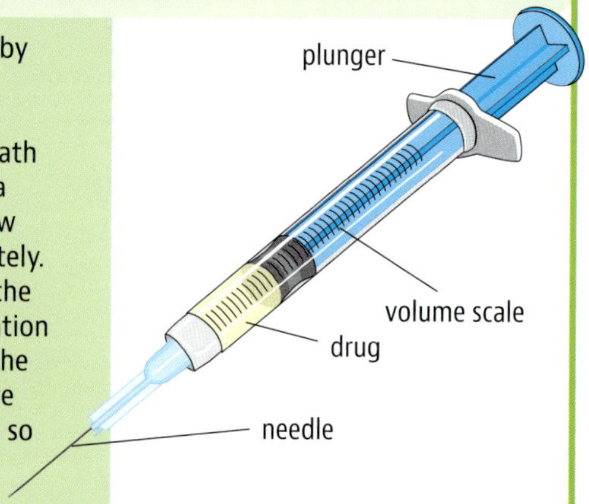

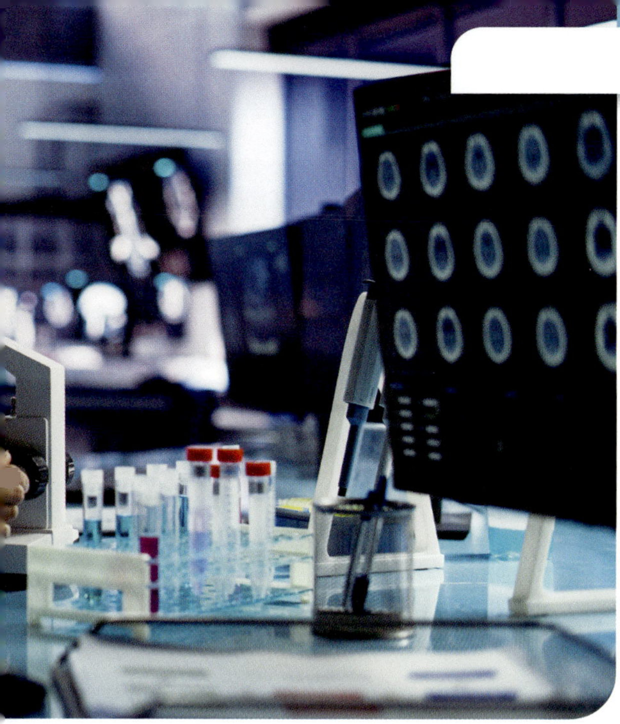

Medical researchers use scientific principles to solve the many mysteries of medicine that still exist, such as the causes of some diseases or the processes of ageing.

PSYCHIATRY AND MENTAL HEALTH

The scientific method was applied to the study of the human mind. Before the 1800s, people were often treated cruelly or just locked up if they showed symptoms of mental illness. French doctor Philippe Pinel (1745–1826) began to classify mental illness and used humane treatment. One of the earliest psychiatrists (from two Greek words for "soul" and "healing") was German scientist Emil Kraepelin (1856–1926). Problems of the mind can range from internalized feelings of depression to violent behavior. There are two common treatments today: For serious problems, drugs may be prescribed; this is usually supplemented by "talking treatment," in which the patient discusses their feelings (and how they deal with them) with a trained, sympathetic therapist.

NURSING PROFESSION

A revolution in nursing also took place during the 19th century, partly due to the work of Florence Nightingale (1820–1910). In 1854, the British public was horrified by news reports of the terrible hospital conditions suffered by soldiers wounded in the Crimean War (1853–1856). Nightingale and a team of 38 nurses were sent to deal with the problem. They saved many lives by improving conditions and care.

When Nightingale returned to England, she opened a training college for nurses at St. Thomas's Hospital in London. Soon nurses were receiving better training, and nursing became a respected profession.

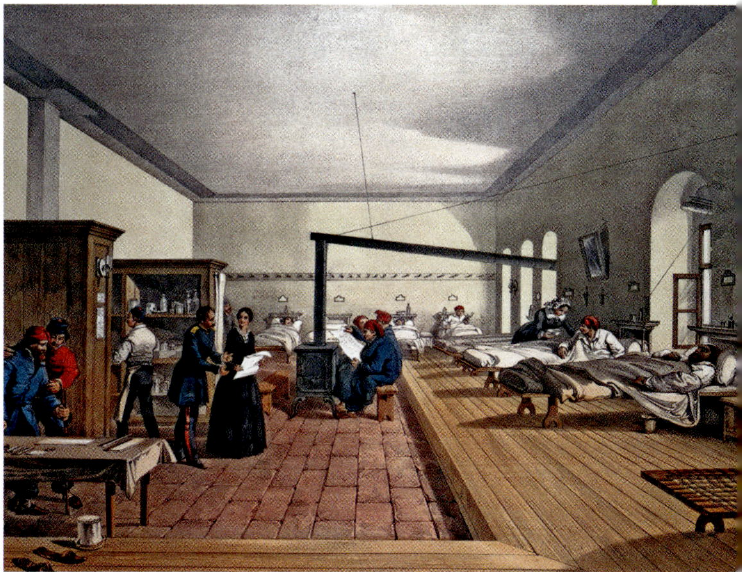

Florence Nightingale became famous for reorganizing the hospital wards in the Scutari Barracks in Istanbul, Turkey, during the Crimean War.

SCIENCE WORDS

Anesthetic: A chemical that stops a patient feeling pain.

Bacteria: Single-celled microorganisms that are present almost everywhere on Earth.

Immunize: To protect from the effects of a harmful substance or disease.

White blood cells: Components of the blood that are responsible for destroying germs and microorganisms.

Fortunately, this was soon to change. In 1799, British chemist Sir Humphry Davy (1778–1829) discovered the anesthetic properties of a gas called nitrous oxide, or laughing gas. When he breathed it in, he found that it made him feel so good that he burst into laughter. It also stopped the pain when he had a tooth pulled out.

Davy suggested that the gas might have medical uses, but his idea was largely ignored. Scientists in the United States, Germany, and France discovered chloroform in 1831, which was also found to be an anesthetic. The liquid was first used by Sir James Young Simpson (1811–1870), a professor of midwifery (the work of helping women with childbirth) in Edinburgh, Scotland. In 1847, he gave chloroform to a woman in labor—the results were so good that in the next week he gave it to another 30 patients. However, other doctors were horrified at his using pain relief in this way because they thought that the pains of childbirth were natural and should not be prevented. Simpson continued to use chloroform, but it was not widely accepted until English Queen Victoria (1819–1901) decided to use it when she gave birth to her eighth child, Prince Leopold.

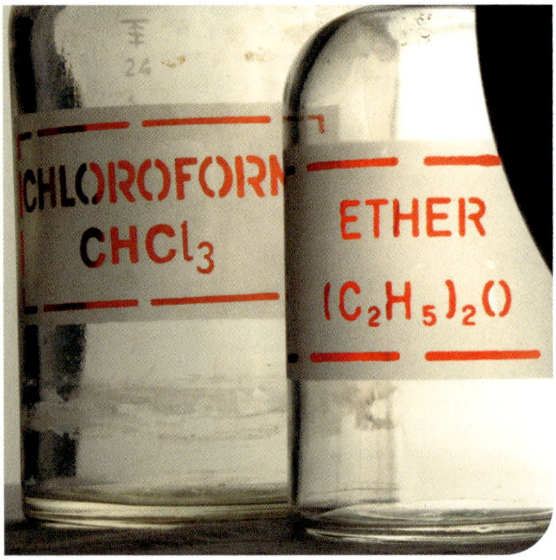

Early anesthetics, such as chloroform and ether, were poured onto a cloth and inhaled from a bowl-shaped mesh held over the face.

Microorganisms and Disease

Bacteriology (the study of bacteria) also began in the 19th century. The idea that microorganisms such as bacteria could cause diseases—the so-called "germ theory"—came about mainly through the work of microbiologists Louis Pasteur (1822–1895) in France and Robert Koch (1843–1910) in Germany.

CHLOROFORM INHALER

The early use of anesthetics was not completely safe. Several patients died from overdoses of chloroform. Junker's chloroform inhaler was invented in 1885 and made anesthetizing patients safer and easier to control. The anesthetic was held in a bottle, and its level could be monitored through a small window. A syringe ball was squeezed to bubble air through the anesthetic. The resulting mixture of air and chloroform vapor passed along a rubber tube to a face mask, which was placed over the patient's mouth and nose. A hook on the inhaler was used for attaching the device to the clothing of the person using it.

SOCIETY AND INVENTIONS

Early Anesthesia

At first laughing gas (nitrous oxide) was used for entertainment at parties in the United States and Britain, but British scientist Humphry Davy suggested that the gas could be used in hospitals for pain relief. Davy's assistant, Michael Faraday (1791–1867), discovered the gas ether, which had a similar effect to laughing gas, and soon people were organizing ether parties. Crawford Long (1815–1878), a surgeon from Atlanta, Georgia, noticed that people felt no pain when they fell over at ether parties. In 1842, he carried out the first operation using ether as pain relief: a boy called James Venable was given the gas before having cysts (lumps) cut from his neck. In 1846, American dentist William Thomas Morton (1819–1868), who was studying medicine at Harvard College at the time, used ether to anesthetize a patient before a surgeon removed a tumor from his neck. The operation was a success. When Robert Liston (1794–1847), a respected British surgeon, heard of this, he used ether on a man who needed his leg amputated. He managed to remove the leg in only 26 seconds. The operation was so painless that the patient was not even aware that it had started.

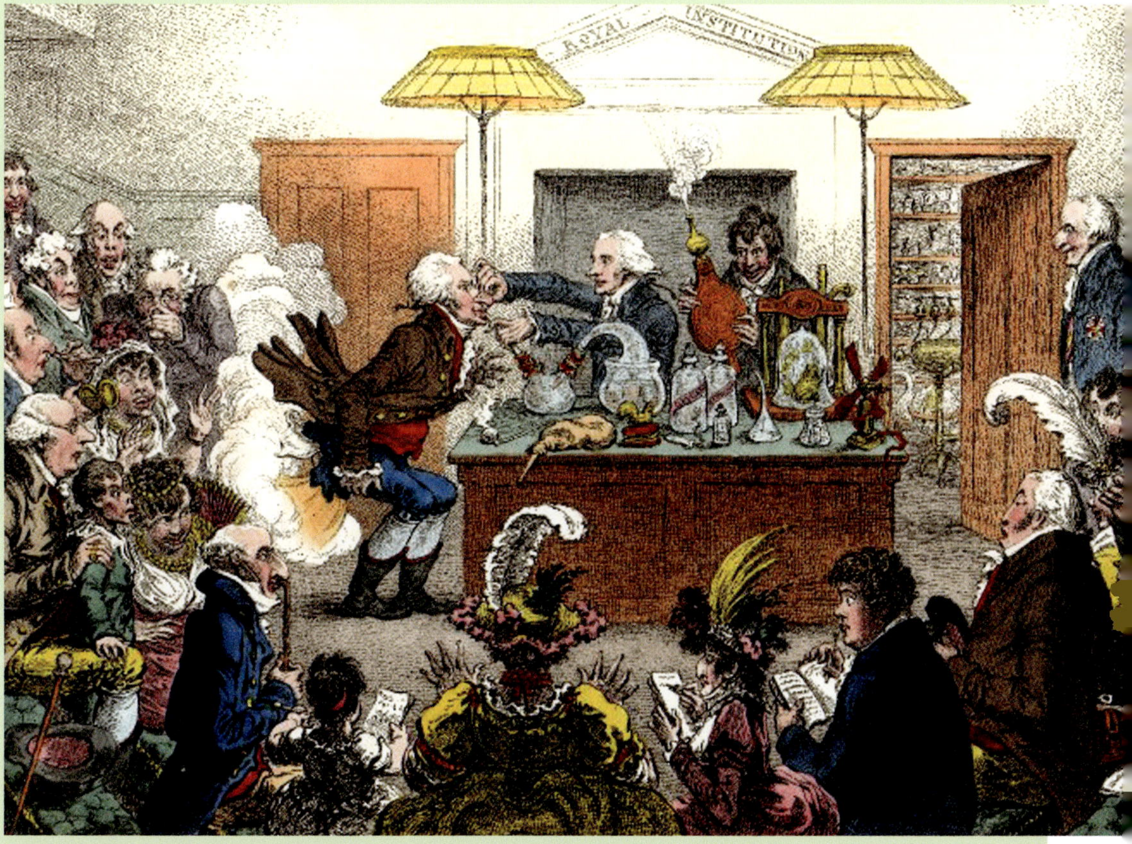

A satirical cartoon shows Humphry Davy (behind the desk, center right, with the bellows) and doctor Thomas Garnett showing off the effects of laughing gas to scientists at London's Royal Institution in 1802.

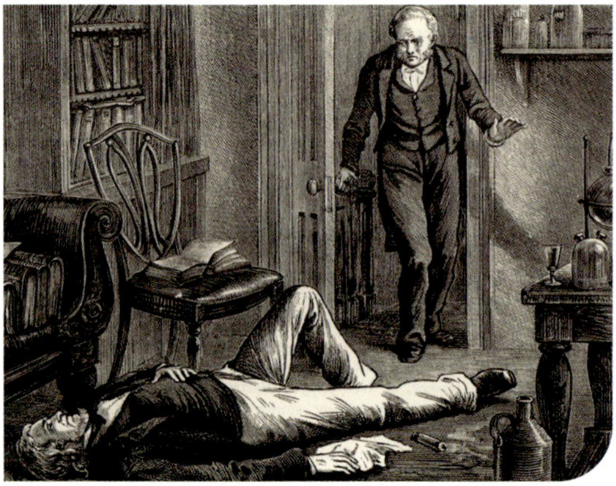

James Young Simpson overcome during an early experiment he was carrying out using chloroform.

While working as a professor of chemistry at the University of Lille during the 1850s and 1860s, Louis Pasteur was asked by the French silk industry to find out why their silkworms were being ravaged by disease. He showed that the disease was caused by a protist (a tiny, single-celled organism) that could be avoided by breeding only with healthy silkworms. Earlier he had demonstrated that some microorganisms cause foods and drinks such as wine and milk to go bad when a process called fermentation goes on too long. As a result of this, Pasteur went on to develop pasteurization, which involves heating and rapidly cooling fresh products (such as milk) to preserve them without cooking them.

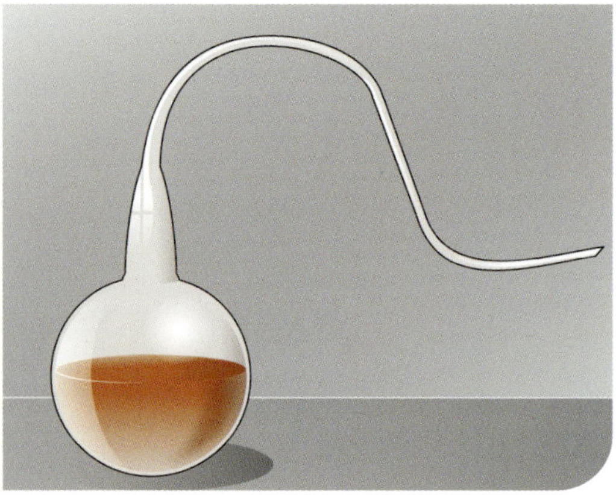

Louis Pasteur used this type of flask in experiments into germs. The sterile broth in the flask stayed fresh because bacteria could not reach it through the swan-shaped neck, while broth exposed to the air soon went sour.

Cause of Disease

Robert Koch went on to show that each disease was caused by one type of microorganism. He found a way of growing bacteria on a solid gel called agar and devised a set of rules that could be used to prove that a particular bacterium was causing a particular disease. In 1876, Koch found that a rod-shaped bacterium causes anthrax (a disease of livestock and humans). He also found the bacterium that causes tuberculosis (a lung disease) in 1882, and the bacterium that causes cholera (a tropical disease that infects the digestive system and is caught by drinking unclean water) in 1883.

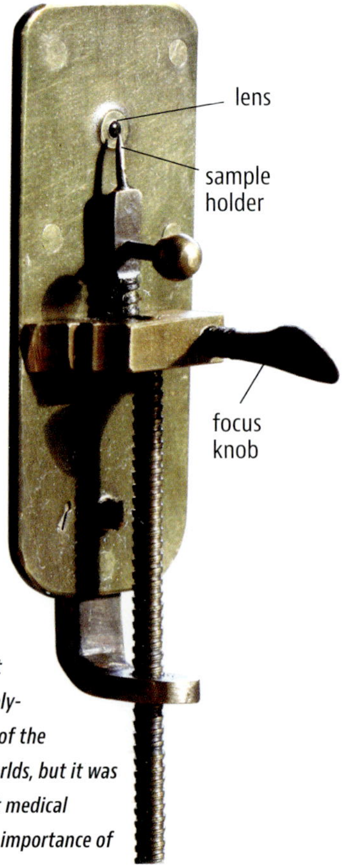

The microscope used by Dutchman Anton Van Leeuwenhoek (1632–1723) in the 1600s. Using this simple device he was the first person to see bacteria and other microorganisms. He kept how he made his lenses a closely-guarded secret. The invention of the microscope opened up new worlds, but it was not until the 19th century that medical science finally understood the importance of microorganisms.

SOCIETY AND INVENTIONS

Defeating Smallpox

At the end of the 18th century, smallpox had replaced plague as the biggest killer. The disease produced disfiguring pustules (sores) all over the body and a large proportion of smallpox sufferers died. However, in China doctors had learned how to give people a weak strain of the disease to protect them against the more deadly illness. By the 18th century, this idea had spread to England.

In the west of England people noticed that dairy maids who caught cowpox (a similar disease) from milking diseased cows seemed to be immune from catching smallpox. In 1774, a farmer called Benjamin Jesty immunized his wife and two sons against smallpox by injecting them with a small amount of pus from an infected cowpox sore. The news of their immunity quickly spread and was heard by a British physician called Edward Jenner (1749–1823). Jenner studied dairy workers for 20 years, and in 1796 he vaccinated eight-year-old James Phipps with cowpox. Six weeks later Jenner infected James with smallpox but the boy did not catch the disease—the vaccine had made him immune.

In 1966 the World Health Organization (WHO) announced that there would be an attempt to wipe out smallpox. More than 600 WHO workers traveled all over the world for 10 years, rushing to outbreaks of the disease. The last person to catch smallpox naturally was a three-year-old Indian girl called Rahima Banu in 1975. Treatment helped her survive. Today, the only surviving virus is kept in a few high-security laboratories.

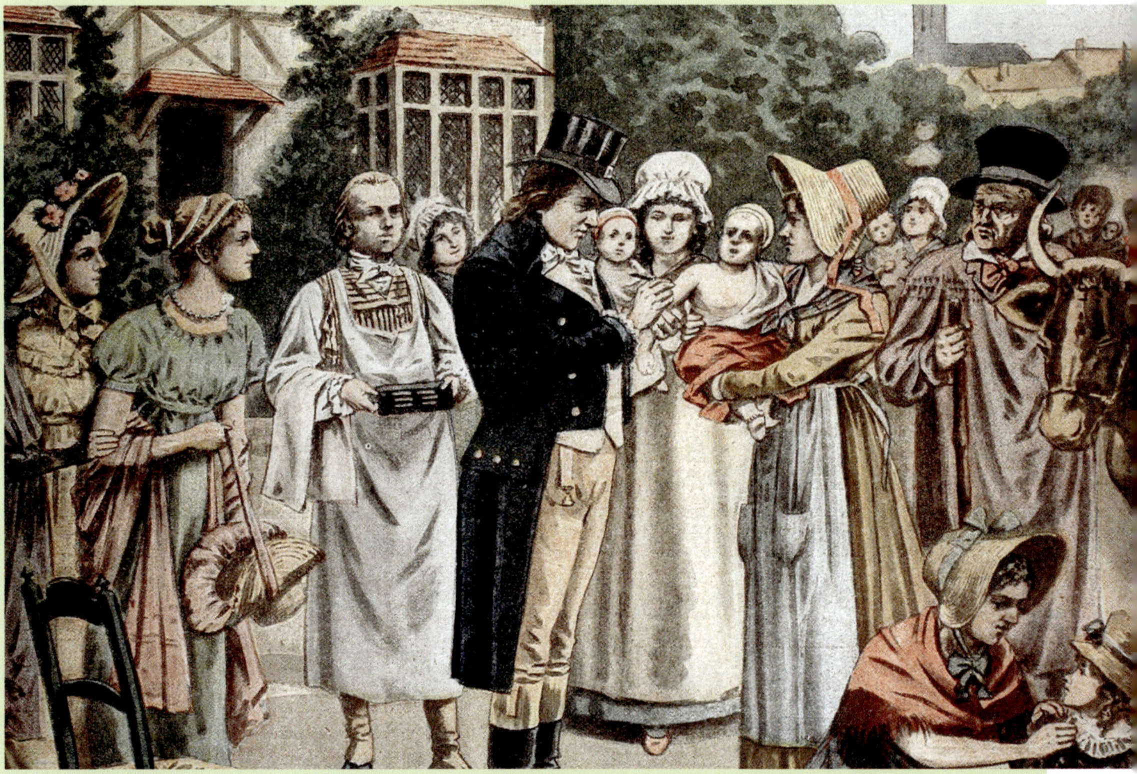

Edward Jenner injects a child with his smallpox vaccine.

FIGHTING INFECTION

Most 19th-century doctors did not appreciate the importance of washing their hands or equipment before treating patients. As a result, open wounds often became infected, leading to amputations. Joseph Lister (1827–1912), a British surgeon who had read Louis Pasteur's work, knew that infection could be reduced by introducing sterile (germ-free) conditions to hospitals.

Lister decided to use carbolic acid as an antiseptic (a substance that kills germs), because it was already used to kill bacteria in sewage. His first antiseptic operation was performed in 1865 on an 11-year-old boy who had suffered a multiple leg fracture after being run over by a cart. Lister washed the wound with carbolic acid and wrapped it in tin foil. Except where the skin was burned by the acid, the leg healed completely. At first, other doctors dismissed Lister's ideas. However, he went on to develop a weaker carbolic acid spray, which he used in 1871 in an operation on Queen Victoria. Eventually, his methods were widely adopted.

While antiseptics made surgery much safer, the harsh chemicals used to kill germs irritated the skin and eyes of the patient, surgeons, and nurses. A better solution was to stop germs from reaching the patient in the first place. This was called aseptic surgery, in which everything in the operating theater had to be thoroughly cleaned before the patient came in. The surgeon's hands and clothes were thoroughly scrubbed. Surgical instruments were placed in a chamber and treated with very hot steam to kill any germs. The sterile gloves, masks, and gowns worn by modern surgeons were invented by the American surgeon William Stewart Halsted (1852–1922).

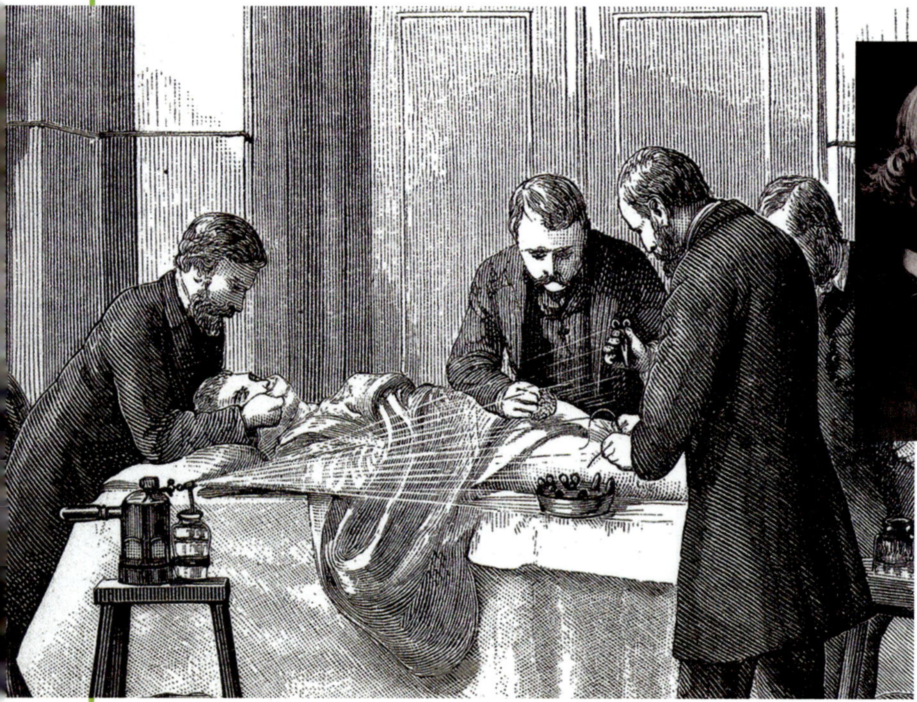

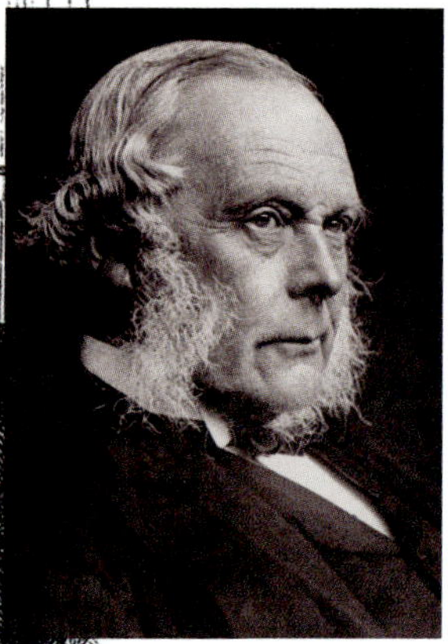

Joseph Lister pioneered his antiseptic techniques in the Glasgow Royal Infirmary in Scotland. He performed surgery in a suit and bowtie.

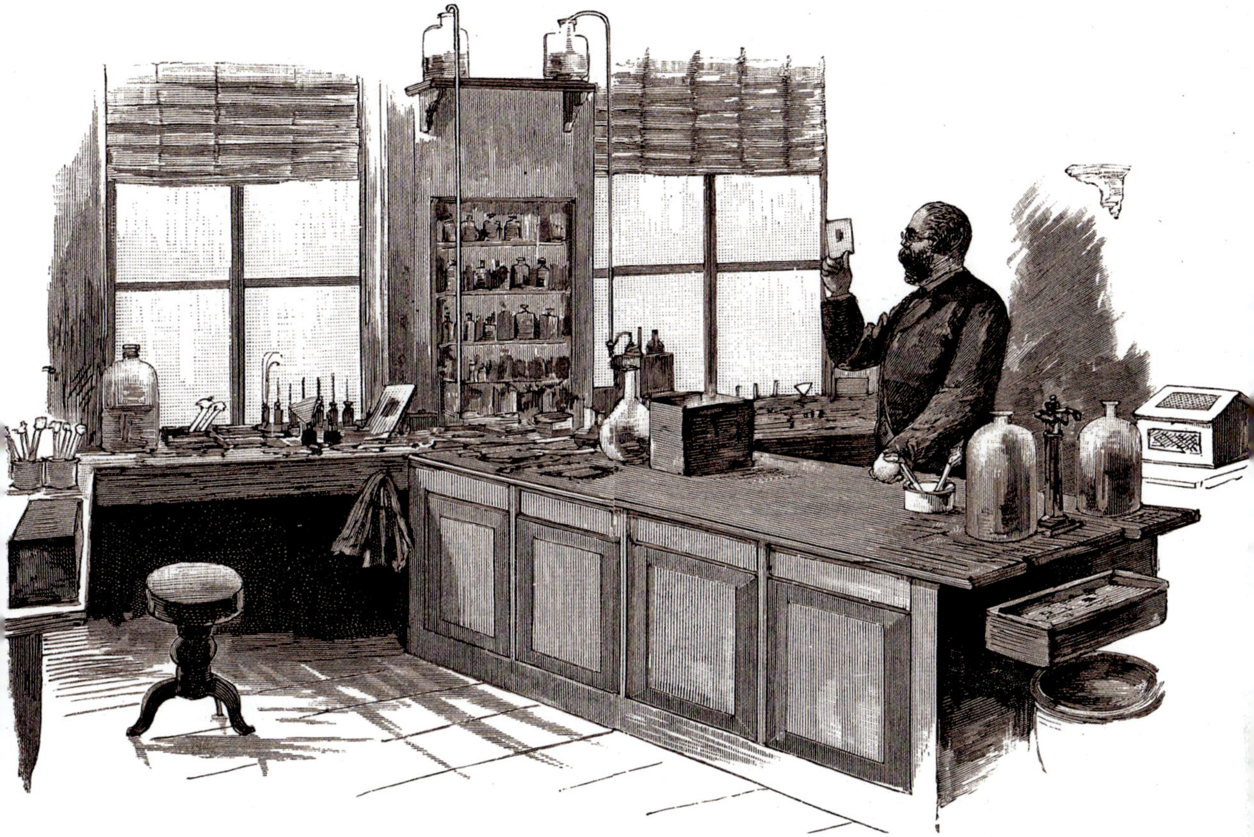

Robert Koch illustrated in his laboratory in the 1890s. His assistant, Julius Petri, invented shallow dishes for growing bacteria samples—known today as petri dishes.

When Louis Pasteur heard about Koch's anthrax experiments, he wondered whether it was possible to immunize (stimulate the body to protect itself) against anthrax. At this time the only disease that could be controlled by immunization was smallpox.

In 1880, Pasteur began research into rabies, a deadly disease of the nervous system. Unfortunately, he was unable to grow the organism that causes it, because it is a virus rather than a bacterium. Despite this problem, Pasteur managed to make a rabies vaccine by injecting rabbits with liquid extracted from

FACTS AND FIGURES

- In 1879, Norwegian doctor Gerhard Armauer Hansen (1841–1912) discovered the bacterium responsible for leprosy, which damages nerves.
- In 1881, plasmodium, a single-celled organism that causes malaria, was discovered by French doctor Alphonse Laveran (1845–1922).
- In 1894, the bacterium that causes bubonic plague was first identified by Swiss-born French microbiologist Alexandre Yersin (1863–1943).
- In 1905, the bacterium responsible for syphilis, a sexually transmitted disease, was discovered by microbiologist Fritz R. Schaudinn (1871–1906).

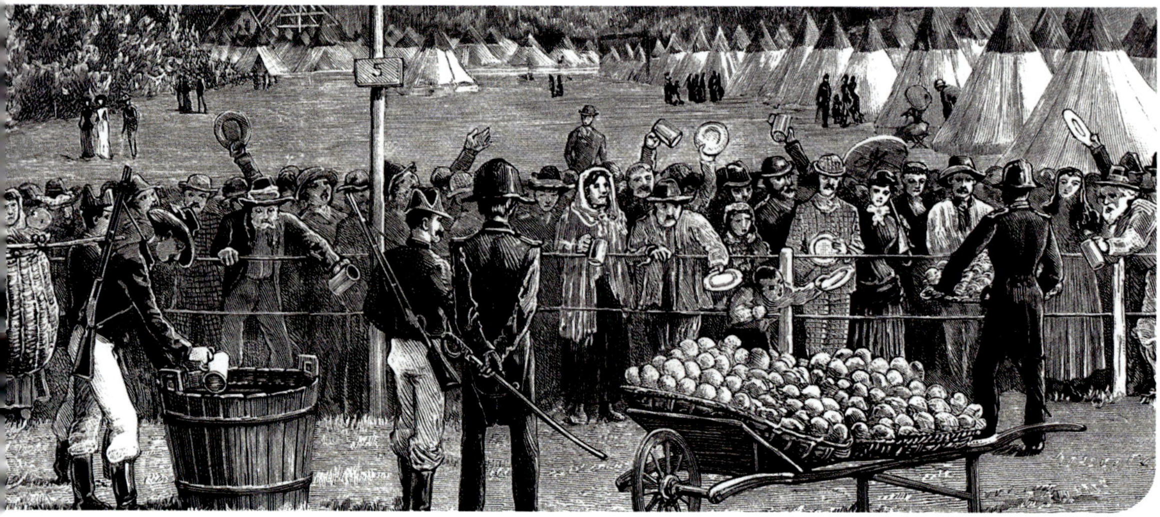

Italian soldiers hold people in a quarantine camp during a cholera epidemic in the 19th century. Doctors had discovered how the disease was spread and the internees were given clean water and fresh fruit.

the spinal cords of diseased animals. When the rabbits died, he dried out the spinal cords to weaken the virus. Although he tested the vaccine on dogs, he was unsure about its safety and reluctant to try it on humans. But in 1885 a nine-year-old boy called Joseph Meister, who had been bitten by a rabid dog, was brought to him. The boy would likely die, so Pasteur tried the vaccine. Treatment took 14 days, and the boy survived. The work of Koch and Pasteur confirmed the germ theory of disease and pointed to methods of combatting germs. The 20th century was to see many more advances.

PASTEUR'S EXPERIMENT

In a famous experiment in 1881, Louis Pasteur injected 24 sheep, a goat, and six cows with his new vaccine, an anthrax bacteria that had been made weak and inactive by growing it at a raised temperature of 108°F (42°C). Two weeks later, Pasteur injected his vaccinated animals and a similar number of unvaccinated animals with active anthrax bacteria. Two days after this, all the vaccinated animals were still healthy, while the unvaccinated animals were dead or dying. Pasteur's fame was sealed by the success of this experiment and confirmed his theory that germs were the cause of many diseases.

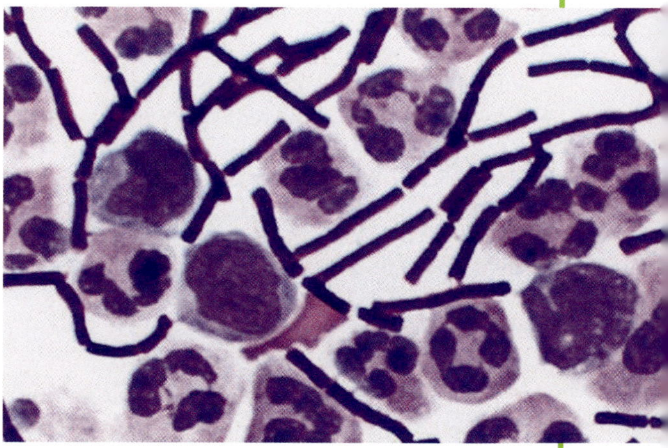

Anthrax bacteria attack livestock, but can also kill people.

VACCINATION

The body is constantly attacked by disease-causing organisms (pathogens) such as bacteria and viruses, which it fights using a process called the immune response. In addition to fighting the pathogen, the body generates memory cells that enable it to detect and destroy the same type of pathogen quicker in the future. Vaccination uses this feature of the immune response:

1 A doctor or nurse injects a vaccine, which is pathogens that have been made harmless in some way, into the patient's bloodstream. A small proportion of the patient's white blood cells have receptors that bind to this pathogen.

2 The white blood cells that have bound to the pathogen divide rapidly into antibody-producing plasma cells and memory cells. The plasma cells release large numbers of antibodies into the blood.

3 The antibodies bind to the remaining pathogens to form clumps, which are absorbed and destroyed by macrophages, another type of white blood cell.

4 The memory cells may remain in the body for many years. If the real pathogen is ever met, they divide more quickly and make even more antibodies than before to destroy it. This is called the secondary immune response.

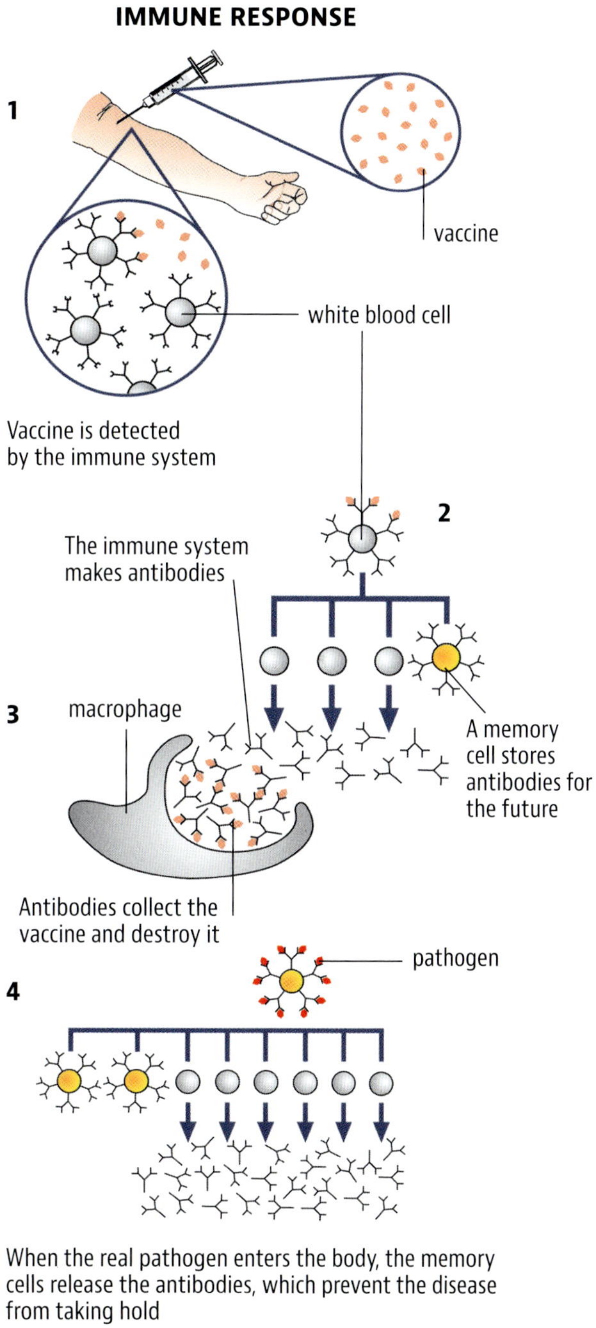

This diagram represents how a vaccine primes the body's natural immunity system to prepare for attack by a disease.

DRUGS

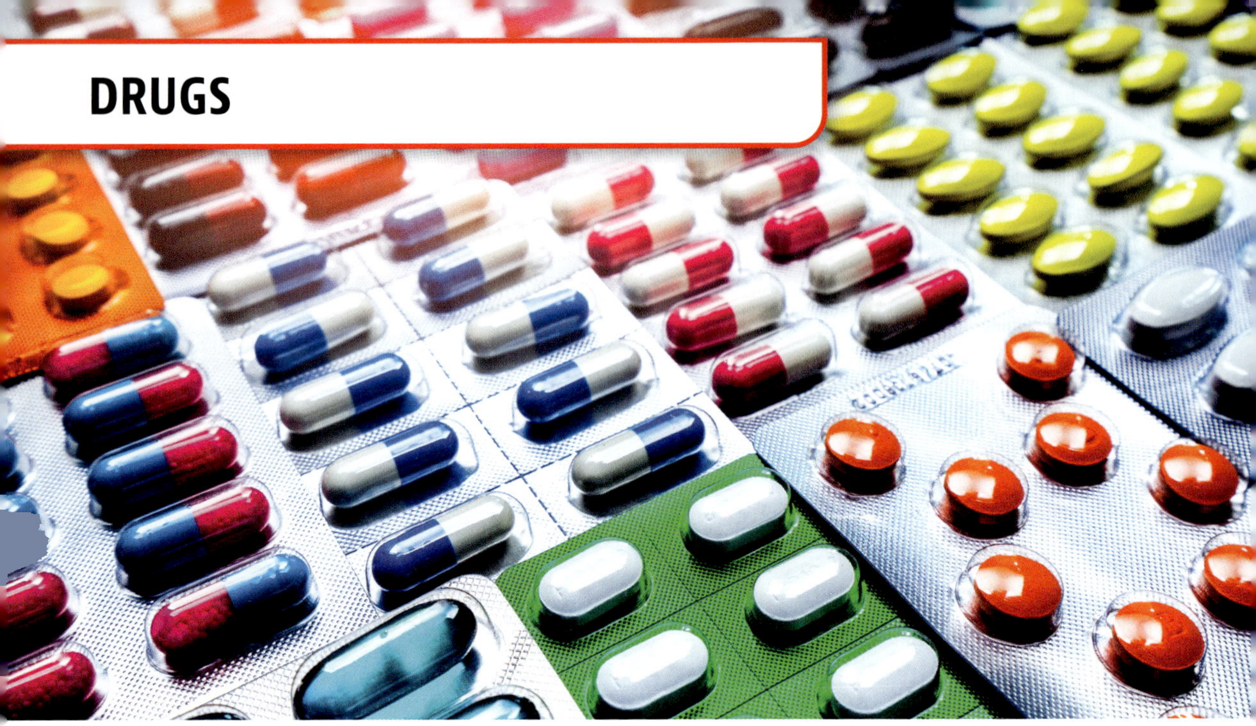

Drugs are substances that have a particular effect on the way the body works, and many kinds can be taken to treat or cure a disease.

Medicines are most easily administered by swallowing pills. The pills are made from harmless chalky substances that dissolve in the stomach, releasing the active ingredients.

Some drugs are found in foods and drinks. Caffeine is a powerful stimulant (something that increases nervous activity in the brain) and a diuretic (something that increases urine flow), and it is found in small but powerful quantities in tea, coffee, and some soft drinks. Alcohol is a drug and can cause serious illnesses. The nicotine in tobacco smoke is a highly addictive drug. Although smoking causes many illnesses, smokers find it hard to stop. Medical drugs are therapeutic: they make the body better. The antibiotic penicillin, for example, can be used to treat infections caused by bacteria. Drugs such as aspirin are taken to relieve pain.

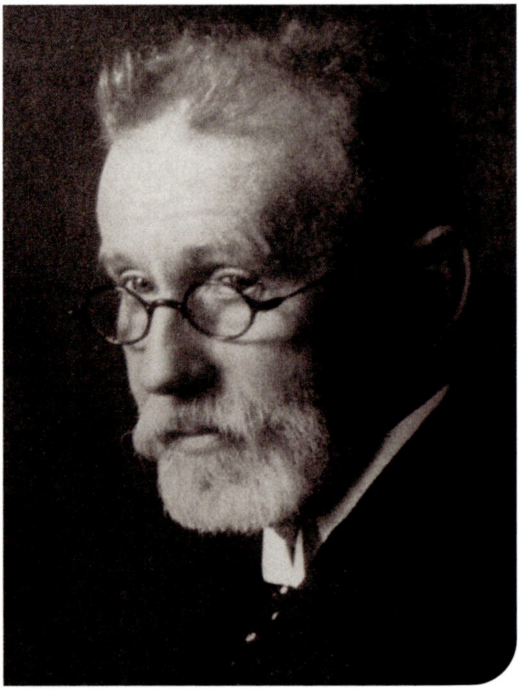

Paul Ehrlich developed the first artificial bacteria-killing drug in the early 20th century.

Magic Bullet

By the 1890s, Paul Ehrlich (1854–1915), a German bacteriologist (a scientist who studies bacteria), had reasoned that it ought to be

THE QUININE STORY

Legend has it that a South American, lost in the high Andes, was burning with fever. He stumbled into a stagnant forest pool and drank his fill of the bitter water to quench his raging thirst. Chemicals from the bark of nearby cinchona trees had leached into the water, giving it the bitter taste. When the man awoke from a deep sleep, his fever had gone. Scientists have since found that the bark of several species of cinchona trees contains a drug called quinine (named for the local name of the tree, *quina-quina*). This drug has become a treatment for malaria, the often-fatal fever-causing disease that is passed on by blood-sucking mosquitoes. Quinine is also the flavoring in the drink known as tonic water.

In the 16th century, Spanish adventurers arrived in South America. They were in search of gold but they ended up finding one of the most useful drugs in modern medicine. The invaders saw that Native Americans chewed cinchona bark to control fever. Spanish Jesuit priests took the tree bark back to Europe in the 1630s, where it became widely used as a malaria treatment. Tonic water was drunk by British colonialists in India and Africa to ward off the disease. It was not until 1820, however, that two French chemists, Pierre Joseph Pelletier (1788–1842) and Joseph Bienaimé Caventou (1795–1877), isolated quinine from the bark of the tree.

During World War I (1914–1918) quinine was used to treat soldiers. At this time supplies to Germany were cut off and so German chemists developed artificial quinine. They devised one form, called quinacrine, and then a better form, called chloroquine. Several other synthetic forms of quinine have since been made. The parasite that causes malaria gradually becomes resistant to most forms of synthetic quinine, however, and new forms have to be found. Quinine, the natural substance, does not encourage resistance in the same way, so it is still an important substance in the battle against malaria.

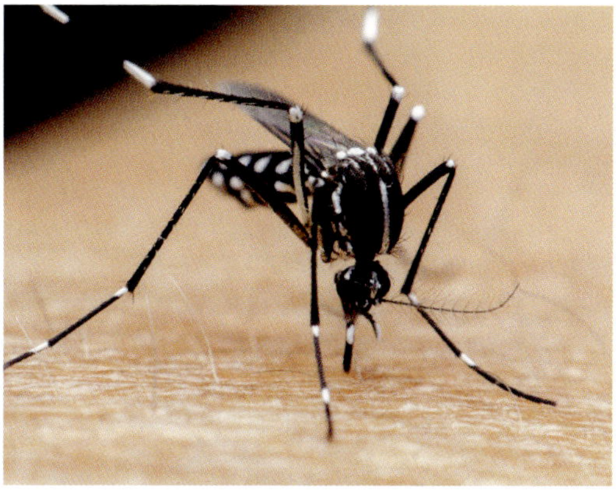

Malaria is spread by the female Anopheles *mosquito, which sucks human blood.*

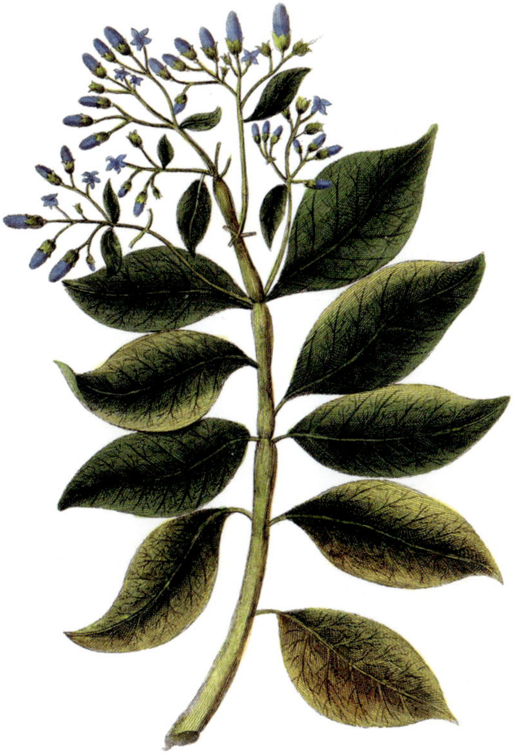

Medicinal chemicals are most concentrated in the bark of cinchona plants. As well as quinine, the plant produces quinidine, used to help unhealthy hearts beat regularly.

HOW MALARIA IS TRANSMITTED

Malaria is caused by several strains of a tiny single-celled parasite called *Plasmodium*. The disease is spread by the bites of female mosquitoes that suck human blood. The best way to protect against malaria is to prevent mosquitoes biting. Mosquitoes are active at night, so sleeping under a net or spreading insect repellents on the skin will stop the insects from biting. Anti-malarial drugs kill the *Plasmodium* if a mosquito does bite.

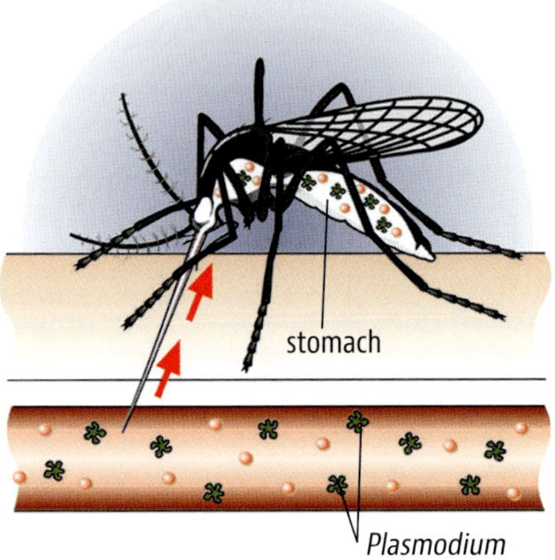

1 A mosquito bites an infected person, picking up some of the malaria parasites with the blood it sucks. The *Plasmodium* multiplies in the mosquito's stomach.

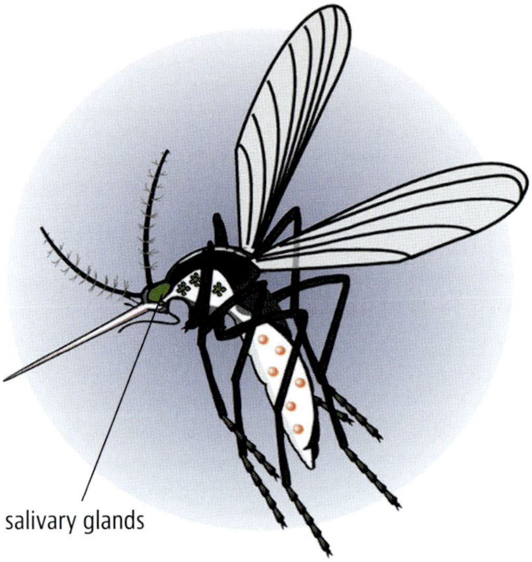

2 The *Plasmodium* migrates to the mosquito's salivary glands.

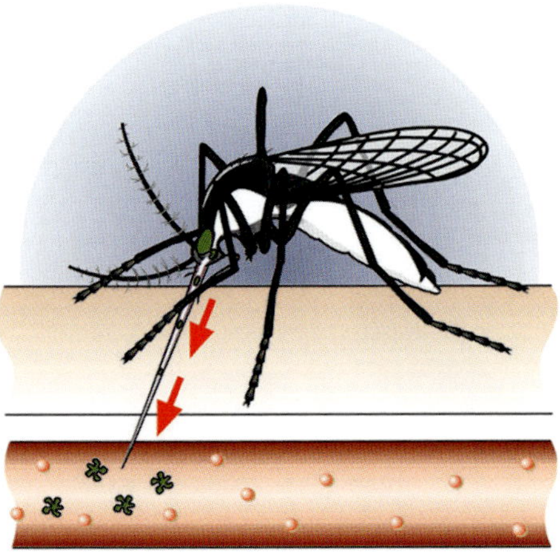

3 When the mosquito bites another person, the *Plasmodium* parasites enter that person's bloodstream along with the mosquito's saliva.

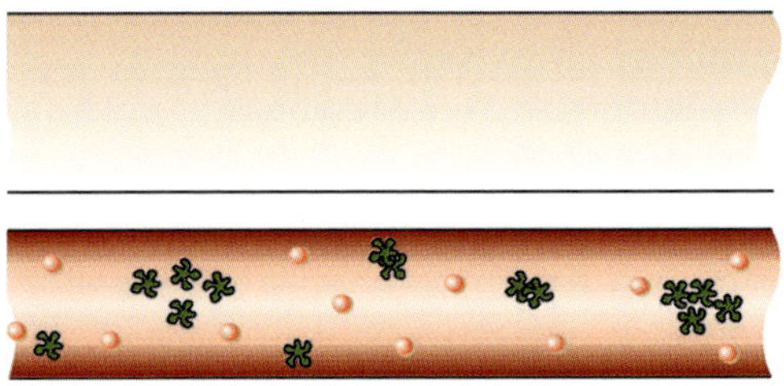

4 The *Plasmodium* travels to the liver, where it multiplies and forms clumps of parasites. These clumps burst and release new *Plasmodium* cells, which invade red blood cells, multiplying again. The red blood cells rupture, causing an attack of fever and releasing even more *Plasmodium* that infect further red blood cells. The cycle of invasion, multiplication, and rupture goes on, causing periodic bouts of high fever.

possible to kill germs that invaded the human body by using certain drugs, if only the right drug could be found. This was the so-called "magic bullet" theory: that a specific chemical could be found that could be used to target a particular kind of cell or microorganism.

Ehrlich was particularly concerned with syphilis, a disease transmitted by sexual contact. He decided to look for a synthetic (artificial) chemical that could be injected into a patient to kill the bacteria that cause syphilis. His Japanese assistant Sahachiro Hata (1873–1938) tested over 600 chemicals before finding the one that worked. This substance was marketed as Salvarsan in 1910, and was the first synthetic "magic bullet." Although Salvarsan did work, it required a series of painful injections before treatment was complete. Taking penicillin tablets was later to prove a much more effective form of treatment for syphilis.

HERBALISM

Drugs have been used for thousands of years. The ancient Chinese practiced herbalism (using plants for medical purposes) over 5,000 years ago. By about 1500 BCE the ancient Egyptians were using tree resins and plant saps to treat many illnesses. Some of these remedies worked, and are still used today, but others, such as giving patients a poisonous herb called hellebore to make them vomit, were harmful. A book written by the ancient Greek physician Pedanius Dioscorides (c. 40–90 CE) mentions more than 500 herbal remedies.

In a period known as the Dark Ages in Western civilization, between about 500 and 1100 CE, progress in medical science happened in Eastern cultures. Islamic doctors added to the list of medicinal herbs found to be useful, and alchemists—the first chemists—found better ways of extracting, purifying, and administering drugs from these herbs so that treatments were more effective. It was not until the 19th century, however, that the use of herbal drugs began to approach being an exact science.

Sulfonamides and Penicillin

In the 1920s and 1930s many scientists looked for other magic bullets that could be used against common, life-threatening, infectious lung diseases such as pneumonia and tuberculosis (TB). Unfortunately, many chemicals that seemed likely candidates proved to be harmful to human cells or did not work well once bacteria had started to multiply inside the body.

SOCIETY AND INVENTIONS

Contraceptive Pill

A group of drugs that has had a big impact on society in the last 50 years are contraceptive pills, often called the "Pill." Taken daily for three or four weeks in every month (depending on the type of pill), they can prevent pregnancy. The Pill was first devised in the late 1950s. It contains synthetic progesterone (progesterone is a hormone that prepares a woman's uterus for pregnancy). The Pill stops a woman releasing eggs from her ovaries. Many experts see the Pill as one of the key factors that led to major social changes in Western societies in the 1960s. A woman's ability to decide whether or when to have children was to have an impact on their ability to have greater control over their lives.

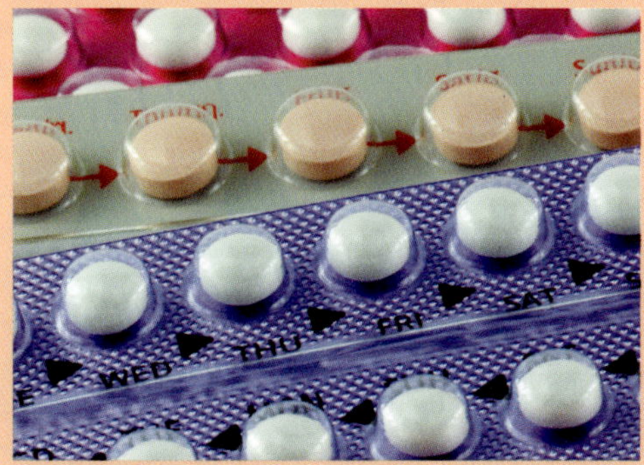

In 1932, German bacteriologist Gerhard Domagk (1895–1964) discovered a red dye called prontosil that killed a bacterium that causes blood poisoning. In the late 1930s, researchers in France, Britain, and the United States developed a range of related drugs called sulfonamides, or sulfa drugs, which were effective against bacterial diseases. These drugs were at the forefront of treatments during the early 1940s, until antibiotics such as penicillin replaced them after World War II (1939–1945).

DRUGS FOR THE MIND

Before the 1950s there were no drugs for treating mental illness. In the late 1940s French surgeon Henri Laborit (1914–1995) was seeking a drug to calm anxious patients just before they had surgery. He found chlorpromazine to be a highly effective drug for the purpose. French psychiatrists Jean Delay (1907–1987) and Pierre Deniker (1917–1998) soon found chlorpromazine to be effective in calming patients suffering from mental illnesses called schizophrenia and bipolar disorder.

Chlorpromazine was the first of half a dozen or so drugs that control extreme behavior, allowing mentally ill patients to leave the hospital and live in the community. By the late 1960s, hundreds of thousands of mentally ill people in North America alone had been successfully released from the hospital under a drug-care program.

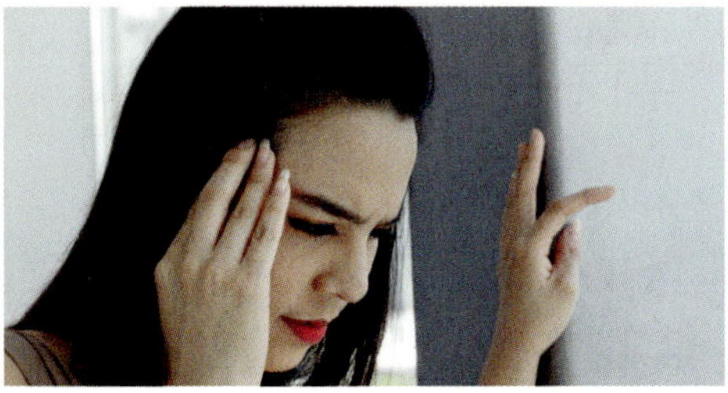

Drugs can change the way people think and how they feel by reducing anxiety or paranoia.

Fleming and Penicillin

British bacteriologist Alexander Fleming (1881–1955) is the famous name linked with the discovery of penicillin, the first antibiotic—a natural substance produced by a fungus that kills or immobilizes bacteria. One day Fleming, looking at some plates used for growing bacteria, noticed that a mold was growing on one of the plates. In an area around the mold there were no colonies of bacteria. It was as if the mold were producing something that was keeping bacteria at bay. In a series of experiments Fleming showed that the *Penicillium* mold produced a substance that could kill the bacteria

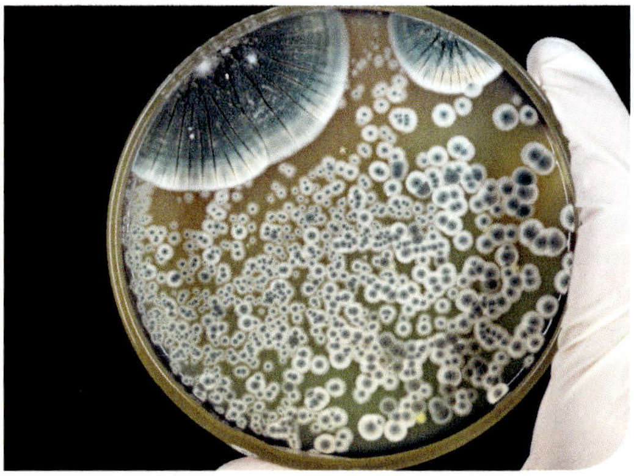

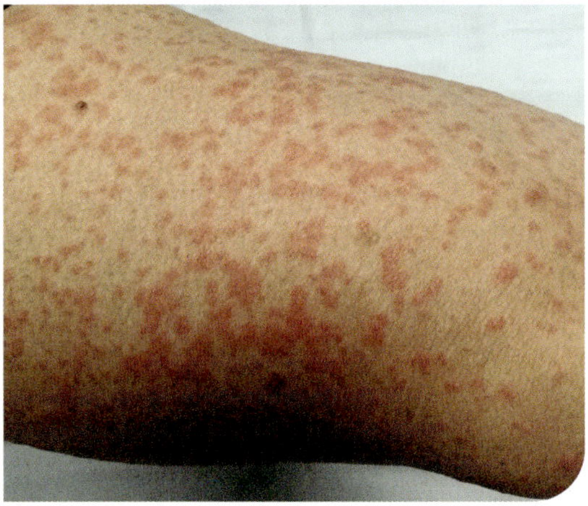

Penicillium *mold growing in a laboratory dish* (top), *and a rash caused by an allergic response to pencillin* (below).

responsible for several common and dangerous bacterial infections, including meningitis (inflammation of the linings and coverings of the brain).

Fleming went on to show that the substance, which he called penicillin, was not harmful to laboratory animals such as mice. He even used some mold extract to successfully treat a colleague's eye infection.

Fleming did not investigate the drug further. That was left to scientists at Oxford University in England led by British biologist Howard Florey (1898–1968) and German-born biochemist Ernst Chain (1906–1979). Between 1939 and 1940 they succeeded in purifying penicillin and testing its effectiveness in mice and people. They could make only tiny

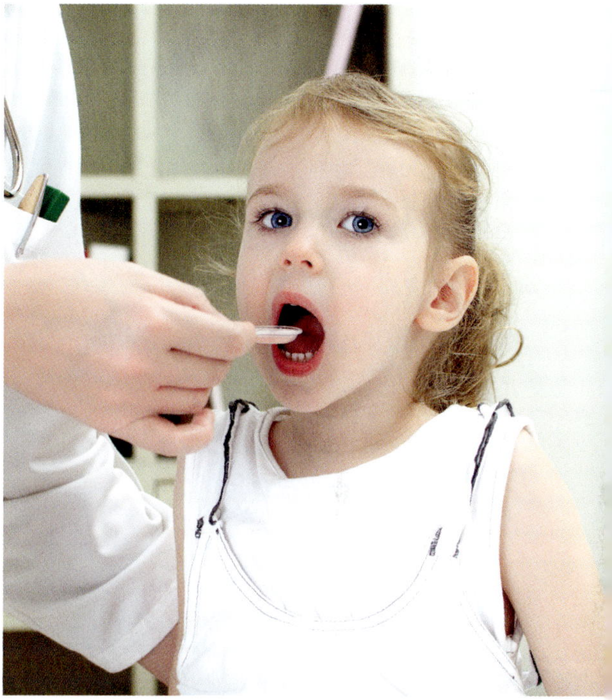

Antibiotics are commonly given to young children as their bodies are more at risk from attack by bacteria.

ANTIBIOTICS

There are two types of antibiotic, each of which has a different way of attacking disease-causing bacteria. Bacteriostatic antibiotics prevent bacteria from growing, which gives the body's immune system time to kill them and eradicate the infection. Bactericidal antibiotics, such as penicillins, actively kill the bacteria.

1 Bactericidal antibiotics destroy bacteria by attacking their protective cell walls. This keeps the cells from maintaining their outer barriers, which then begin to disintegrate.

2 This allows water to flood into the bacteria.

3 The water causes the bacteria to swell and explode.

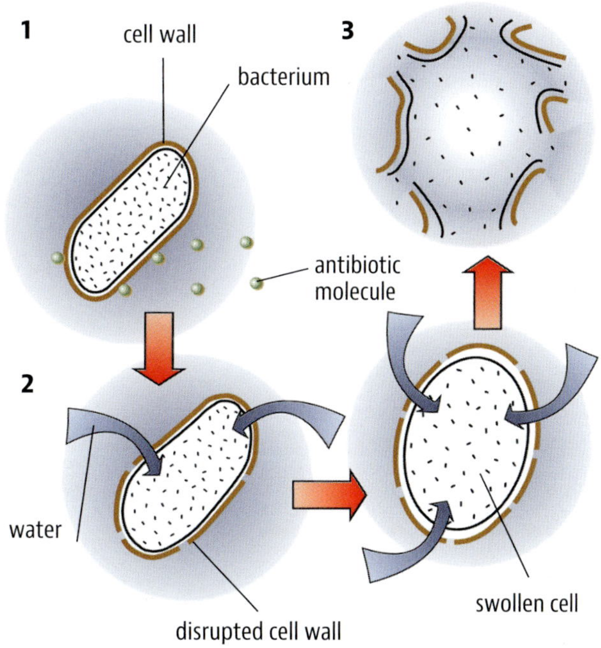

quantities of the drug, however. Money and resources were scarce because it was wartime. Florey and Chain went to the United States to get the funds they needed to make penicillin in large quantities. Toward the end of the war in Europe, in 1944, there were sufficient supplies of penicillin to treat all the injured Allied soldiers. After 1945, it came into general use for civilians.

Penicillin was soon found to be effective against a wide range of bacteria, including those common forms that caused blood poisoning. Dozens of other antibiotics have since been found in all kinds of microorganisms, and new ones have also been manufactured artificially. However, there is a down side to this treatment. Antibiotics have been used in such a widespread manner—even routinely being put in animal feed to prevent farm animals getting infections—that many bacteria are now resistant to some antibiotics. Scientists have to find or devise new antibiotics to keep one step ahead of the microorganisms. If they cannot, there is a serious danger that medicine will be returning to the days before antibiotics existed and there was nothing to kill the most dangerous bacteria.

FACTS AND FIGURES

- Aspirin was the first truly synthetic drug, developed in the 1890s.
- It is used to fight pain and swelling, to lower fever, and to thin the blood (which helps prevent heart attacks). It is thought it may even help prevent bowel cancer.
- In 1997, doctors found that on very rare occasions aspirin caused Reye's Syndrome, a brain disorder in children. As a result, children under 16 should not be given aspirin.

Killing Pain

As well as tackling disease, many drugs have been developed for treating everyday pain, such as headaches, toothache, and arthritis (inflammation of the joints). In the 1820s, Swiss scientist Johann Pagenstecher (1783–1856) found a painkilling substance—

Meadowsweet produces a natural version of aspirin.

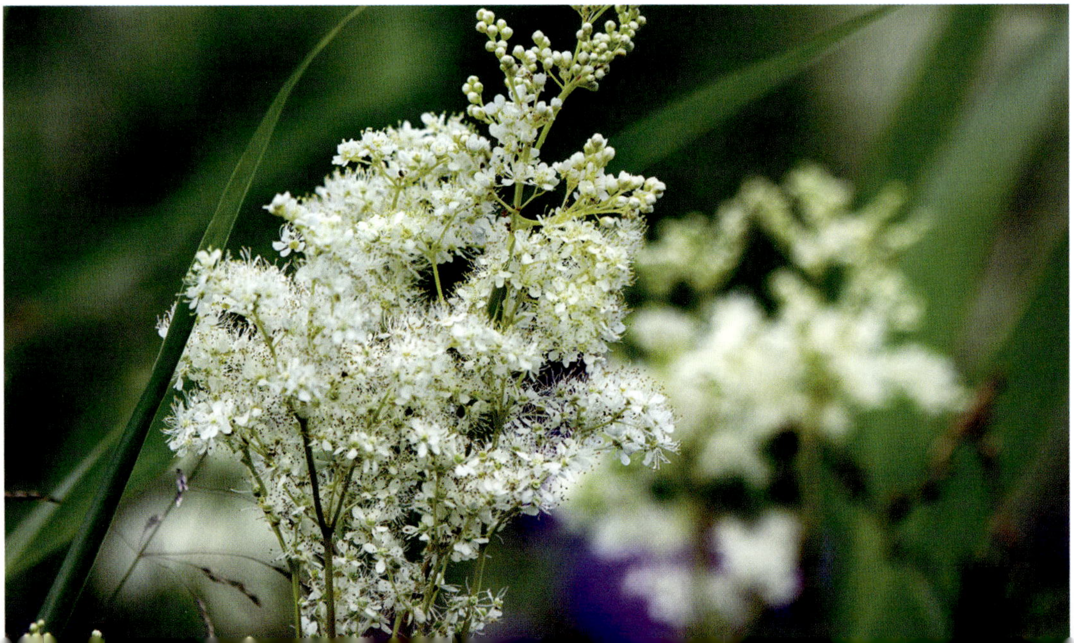

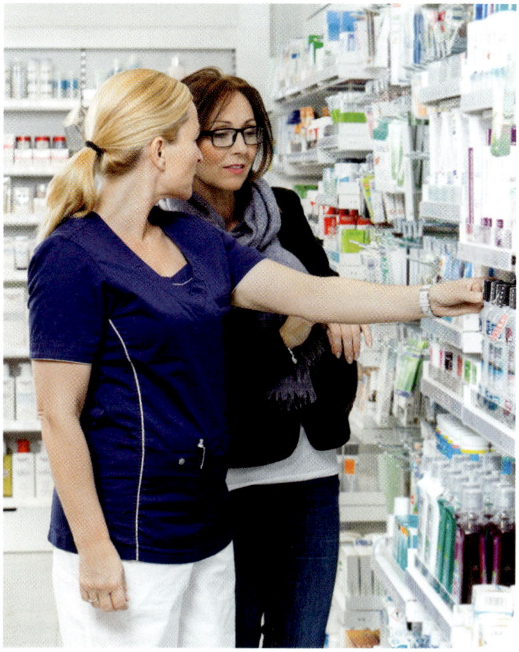

Drugs such as aspirin, paracetamol, and ibuprofen, which ease headaches and other minor pains, are available at drugstores.

later described as salicylic acid—in the meadowsweet plant. The structure of this new drug was discovered in 1853 by Charles Frédéric Gerhardt (1816–1856), a chemistry professor at Montpellier University in France. Unfortunately, it badly irritated the stomach lining and was only used by people whose pain was so severe that the side effects would be acceptable.

One user was Herr Hoffman, who lived in Germany and had severe arthritis. His son, Felix Hoffman (1868–1946), was a chemist at the Bayer Drug Company, and he decided to change the drug to help his father. He came up with a new drug called acetylsalicylic acid, which gave his father his first pain-free night in years. In 1899 this drug was given the name aspirin. Aspirin was the most widespread painkiller available to buy over the counter until the 1980s, when acetaminophen, also known as paracetamol, overtook its sales.

THE THALIDOMIDE TRAGEDY

In the 1950s, Wilhelm Kunz, a chemist working at Chemie Grunenthal in Germany, invented a substance called thalidomide, which seemed to be the ideal sleeping tablet. It worked well and seemed to have few, if any, side effects. However, in the late 1950s reports of side effects began to appear. In 1961, Australian physician William McBride reported the news that some pregnant women who had taken thalidomide in early pregnancy had given birth to children with deformed arms and legs. By the end of 1962, the drug had been withdrawn, but not before 7,500 thalidomide children had been born worldwide.

The episode triggered a worldwide strengthening of the procedures for testing new drugs. In the United States, an important drugs amendment was passed by Congress in 1962. In 1989 the drug was shown to exist in two forms, one that has the sedative (sleep-inducing) effect and the other that is responsible for birth defects. Thalidomide is now used, under carefully controlled conditions, for treating Hansen's disease (also known as leprosy, an infection that causes nerve damage), certain forms of cancer, and immune disorders (malfunctions of the body's defense system).

The Search for New Drugs

Drug companies use four main methods in their search for the wonder drugs of the future. The first is to imitate or use a natural substance that is already believed to be useful. Today there are few opportunities for this because the majority of traditional remedies have already been studied. A second approach involves copying an existing drug but changing its design slightly in the hope of making it even better. A third approach is to design tailor-made drugs, working from knowledge about how the body works. The fourth method is simply to screen thousands of organisms for medically useful chemicals. Today drug companies scour tropical rainforests and coral reefs in search of plants and animals containing unusual chemicals that could be used in medicine. However, finding such substances yields both a promise and a threat. If an anticancer drug is found in a coral reef sponge, for example, and the chemical proves to be effective, there is then the problem of how to produce the drug in large quantities without driving the sponge to extinction.

Devising synthetic chemicals that are similar to natural ones is often seen as the way forward. An alternative is to use genetic engineering techniques in which one easily grown organism produces the chemicals needed. Increasingly effective drugs are being developed for diseases such as AIDS and cancer, and gene-therapy (where genes are modified or "edited") will provide cures for genetic (inherited) diseases.

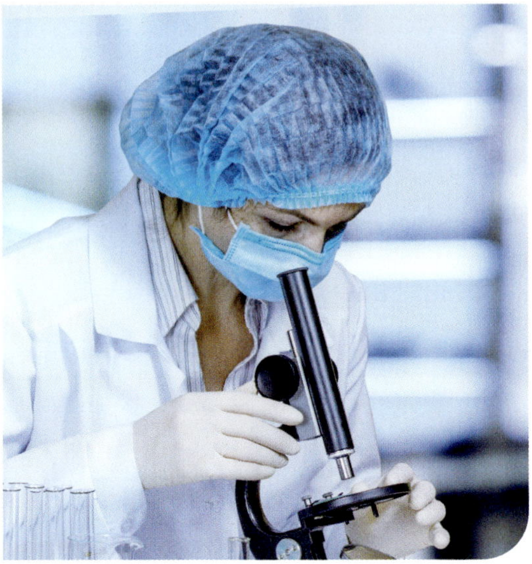

Working with substances with unknown effects is risky, so researchers protect themselves from exposure.

New drugs are tested on animals before they are given to human subjects. Blood tests and other observations are taken to check if the drug is causing harm or distress.

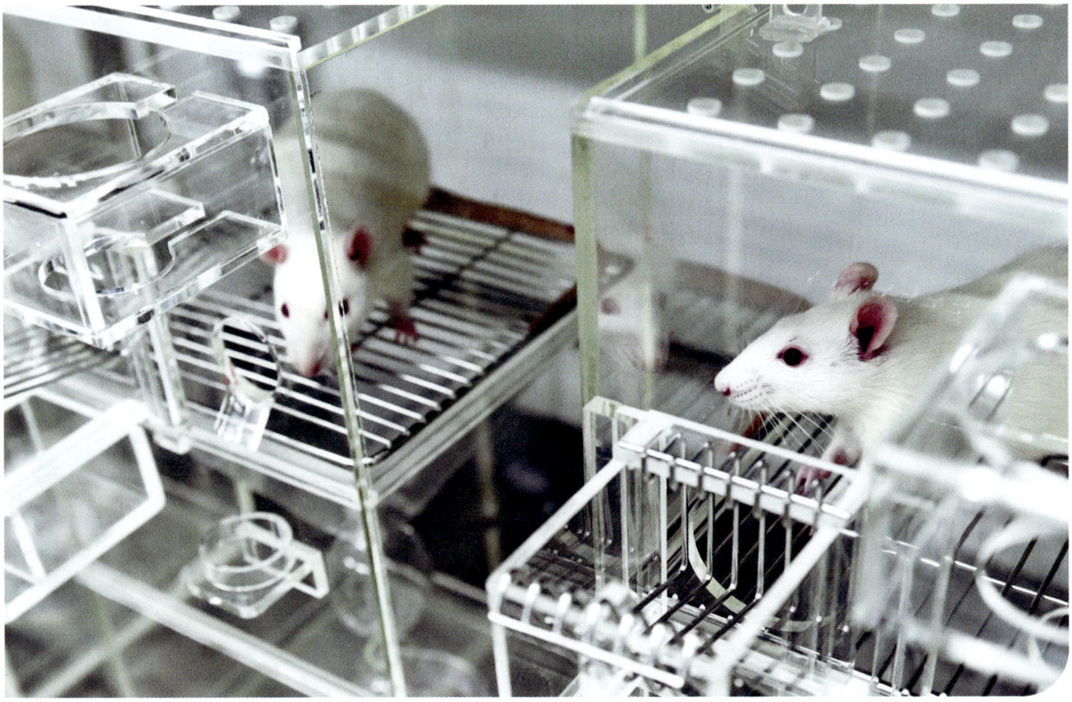

A HOSPITAL PHARMACY

This table lists some of the drugs found in a typical hospital. They are in a variety of forms: tablets dissolve in the digestive system, and their active ingredients are absorbed by the body. Injections are used for more immediate or local effect. Sprays, inhalers, creams, and suppositories are also used.

TYPE	ROLE	ACTION
Analgesics 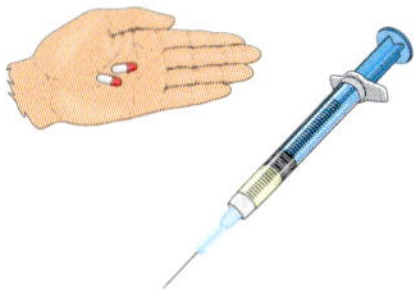	• Nonnarcotic analgesics (such as aspirin and ibuprofen) give short-term relief of moderate pain. • Narcotic, or opiate, analgesics (such as codeine and morphine) give short- or long-term relief of severe pain.	• Stop the pain response at the sites of inflammation. • Suppress the brain's ability to register pain but also cause sleepiness.
Anesthetics 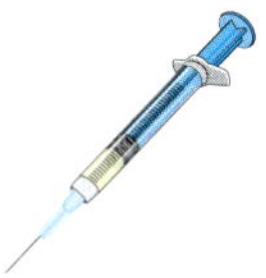	• General anesthetics eliminate all sensory perception, so patients can undergo major operations while unconscious, feeling no pain. • Local anesthetics eliminate sensory perception in one area, allowing, for example, a dentist to painlessly extract a tooth.	• General and local anesthetics suppress the nervous system. 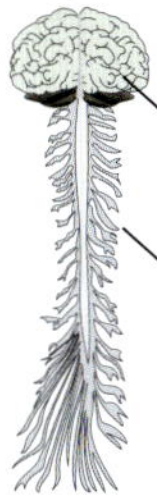
Antibiotics and sulfa drugs 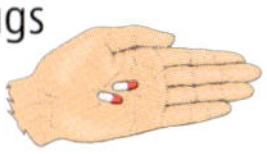	• Fight bacteria that cause diseases.	• Antibiotics work either by killing bacteria or by preventing them from multiplying.
Antitumor drugs 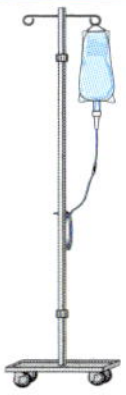	• Treat cancers (unrestrained growth of cells), for example, after surgery to remove a tumor or during chemotherapy (the treatment of cancer using drugs). 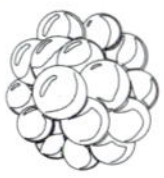	• Antitumor drugs kill all cells that are dividing, including cancer cells but also healthy cells, for example, in bone marrow, giving these drugs considerable adverse side effects.
Depressants 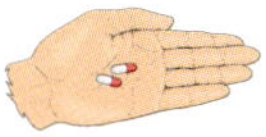	• Tranquilizers reduce tension and worry. • Sedatives make people sleepy.	• Depressants decrease activity of the nervous system but can be addictive.
Immunosuppressant drugs 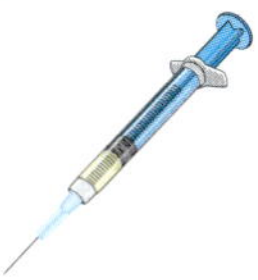	• Prevent autoimmune disorders in which people's white blood cells—their immune system—attack harmless cells in the body, causing damage. • Help prevent rejection of transplants.	• Immunosuppressants interfere with the production and activity of white blood cells, and so they can also increase the risk of infection and the development of cancers.

DIAGNOSIS AND TESTING

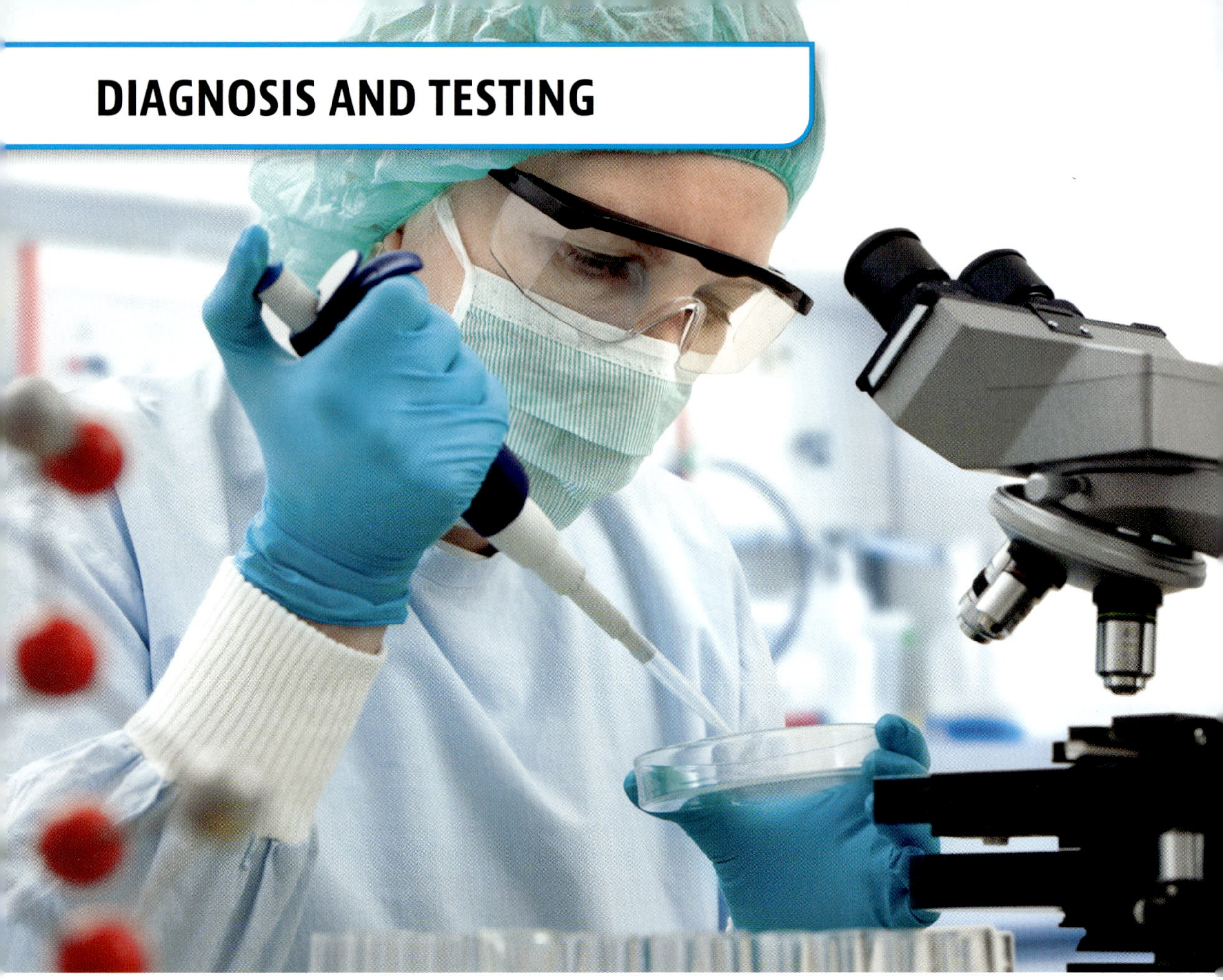

Diagnosis is the process of deciding the nature and cause of a person's ill health. In ancient times diagnosis was largely hit-and-miss Today, diagnosis and testing is a much more accurate science.

By 400 BCE, Chinese medical practitioners were trained in the art of diagnosis. In diagnosing an ailment, Chinese physicians first felt for pulses—six in each wrist. Doctors thought illness was an imbalance between two forces called the yin (dark, moist energy) and the yang (bright, dry energy). Medical conditions were often treated with acupuncture, in which thin needles were inserted into specific points on the body, and herbalism, which was the use of plants.

In medieval Europe ideas about diagnosing and treating disease had changed little from ancient Greek and Roman times. The theory of the four humors was still used as a framework for diagnosis, although it had now changed into the theory of complexion, or temperament. A person with too much black bile, for example, was melancholic (sad or depressed). As in Greek and Roman times, diagnosis could take time.

European physicians would listen to their patients' stories, feel for the pulse, and sometimes make a detailed physical examination. Treatments included being given herbal remedies to make the person vomit and get rid of black bile, or controlled bleeding to draw off blood and so restore the balance of the humors.

SOCIETY AND INVENTIONS

Body in Balance

Doctors in ancient India thought that the body consisted of four substances. These were blood (rakta), phlegm (kapha), bile (pitta), and wind (vayu). All diseases were caused by imbalances of these mysterious substances. By the third century BCE this idea, along with others from the early Egyptians, was modified by the ancient Greeks in their theory of the four humors. Greek doctors thought a person's health resulted from the balance of the humors corresponding to the four basic elements of nature: blood carried air; yellow bile was filled with fire; black bile contained earth; and phlegm was full of water. Each humor had particular properties. Phlegm was linked with cold and damp. Too much phlegm, brought on by cold weather, was thought to cause colds and flu.

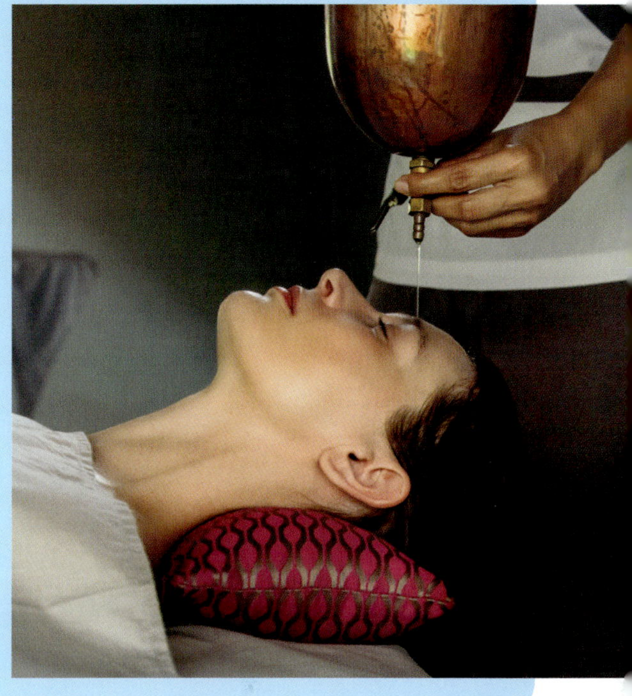

Warm oil is trickled on the head during an Indian head massage. It is meant to relax and rebalance the elements within the body.

SOCIETY AND INVENTIONS

Diagnosing Illnesses

Today's doctors have advanced medical technology, helping them to make accurate diagnoses. Tissue samples can be taken and viewed through high-power microscopes. Specimens of many kinds can be taken, and any microorganisms they contain grown for identification. Body fluids can be analyzed for their detailed chemistry, and the body itself can be scanned. Artificial intelligence (AI) is helping doctors diagnose diseases early. AI can analyze large amounts of information quickly and accurately. This means that illnesses can be diagnosed and treated at an early stage, leading to better outcomes. However, technology will never entirely replace a doctor's human touch.

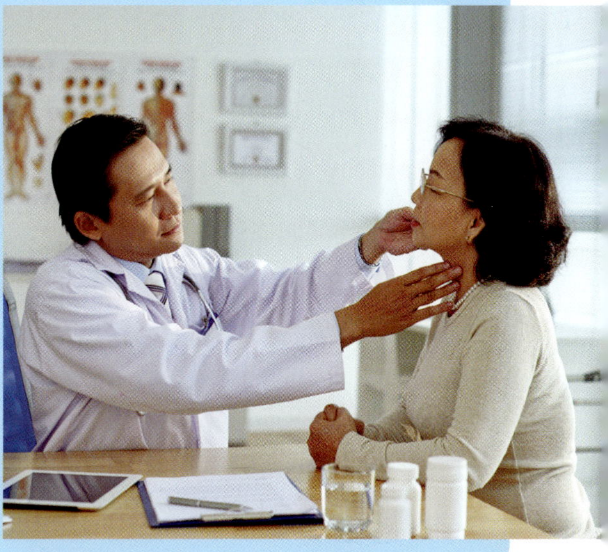

Just looking and touching may tell a doctor if a sore throat needs treatment.

Slow Development

More sophisticated forms of diagnosis were slow in coming. It was only in the 17th century that the first microscopes were made. The early ones, such as those used by Italian biologist Marcello Malpighi (1628–1694), professor of medicine in Pisa, Italy, could show the tiny blood vessels called capillaries.

WAVE DETECTION

By the early 20th century, scientists and physicians were eager to measure any physical and chemical features of the body that might prove useful in diagnosing damage or disease. In 1903 Dutch scientist Willem Einthoven (1860–1927) performed the first electrocardiograph (ECG). This was a recording of the electrical activity of the heart. The device he used, called a string galvanometer, was bulky, but by 1928 portable machines were being used that weighed only 30 lb (14 kg). In the 1920s German biologist Hans Berger (1873–1941) used a string galvanometer to detect brain waves. This led, by the early 1940s, to electroencephalograms (EEGs). These are recordings of brain activity used to diagnose epilepsy and detect brain injuries.

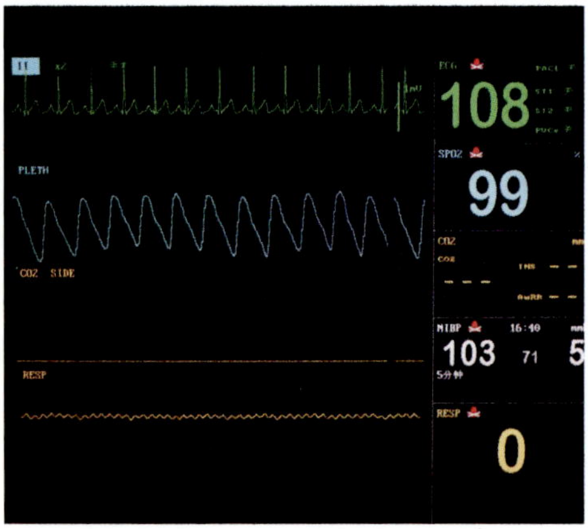

The electrical activity of a heart can be analyzed on computer, displayed on a screen, and then printed out.

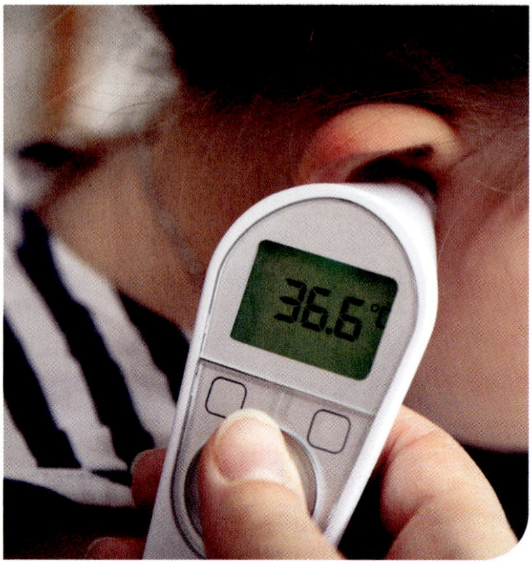

A doctor measures the temperature of a patient using a digital thermometer placed in the ear. This gives an accurate reading in just a few seconds.

However, it was still nearly 200 years before the pioneering work of French chemist and microbiologist Louis Pasteur (1822–1895) and German bacteriologist Robert Koch (1843–1910) would identify specific microorganisms such as bacteria and protists (tiny, single-celled organisms) seen through a microscope, and link them to particular diseases.

Another problem in diagnosis at the time was a general lack of knowledge about body chemistry. The best way to diagnose many conditions was later found to be by analyzing substances in the body. Protein in urine, for example, could be a sign of kidney problems. However, at the end of the 18th century chemistry was still in its infancy.

Signs and Symptoms

Despite limitations in making diagnoses, European medicine had become much more scientific by the end of the 18th century. Doctors were carrying out experiments, made detailed observations, and kept careful records of a patient's signs (what the doctor can see or measure) and symptoms (what the patient is able to tell the doctor about how they feel).

Thermometers

The clinical thermometer is an important piece of medical equipment. It is used to measure the body temperature of a patient. Various Italian scientists developed bulky thermometers in the late 16th century. Santario (*see page 5*) was one of these; Galileo Galilei (1564–1642) was another. In the early 18th century, German physicist Daniel Gabriel Fahrenheit (1686–1736) devised his temperature scale. However, it was not until 1867 that British physician Thomas Clifford Allbutt (1836–1925) developed the first small mercury thermometer that registered quickly and accurately. Before this, standard thermometers were more than 12 inches (25 cm) long and took 20 minutes to register. Measuring body temperature soon became a standard medical examination. A raised temperature was seen as a clear sign of fever, which is a common symptom of many diseases.

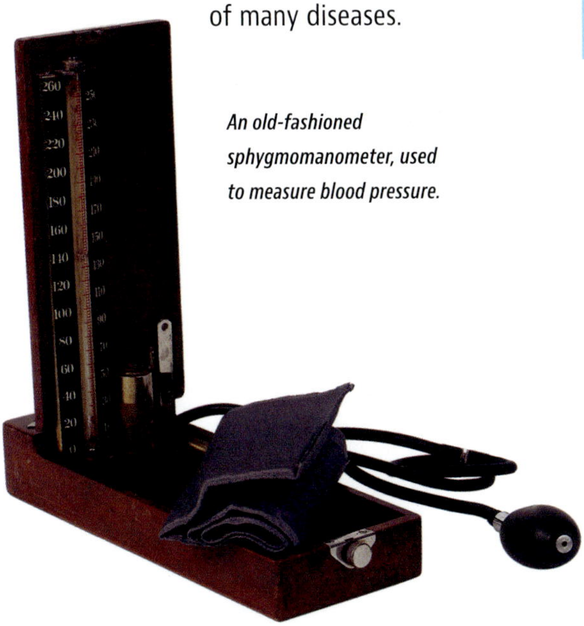

An old-fashioned sphygmomanometer, used to measure blood pressure.

ENDOSCOPES

An endoscope is an instrument that is passed into the body through an opening, such as the nose or throat. An early version was used in 1826, when French doctor Pierre Ségalas (1792–1875) designed a hollow, metal tube, or speculum, so that he could see inside the bladder. The procedure became routine in the 1950s, when fiber-optic technology was developed. By 1965, Professor Harold Hopkins (1918–1994) had devised an endoscope that produced clear, magnified images.

Modern endoscopes are long and flexible, and contain hundreds of tiny glass strands (fiber optics) that carry light to the tip. The tip may contain a camera that transmits pictures to a screen. The tips are equipped with tiny surgical instruments so they can take tissue samples to aid diagnosis. Scissors cut through tissue and remove growths, brushes take samples of cells for analysis, and lasers burn off growths. Water-and-air-supply tubes allow the doctor to wash and dry the tissues that are being looked at. Endoscopes may also be used to carry out surgery. This type of operation—called keyhole, or noninvasive, surgery—minimizes damage to surrounding tissues and allows patients to recover much more quickly than after normal surgery.

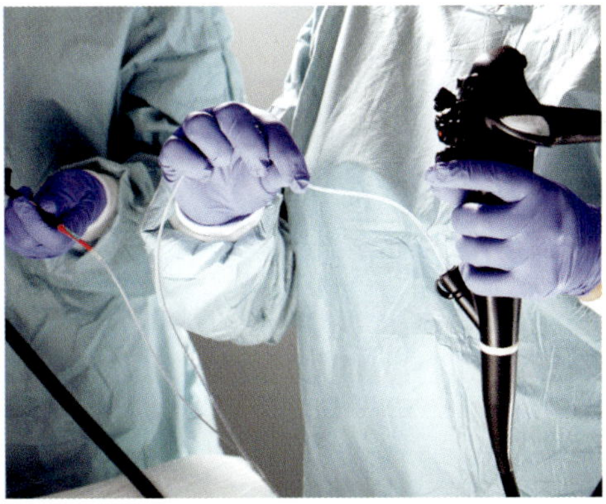

A surgeon feeds a drainage tube into an endoscope. The handle of the device has several grips and switches for controlling the tool at the end of its flexible tip.

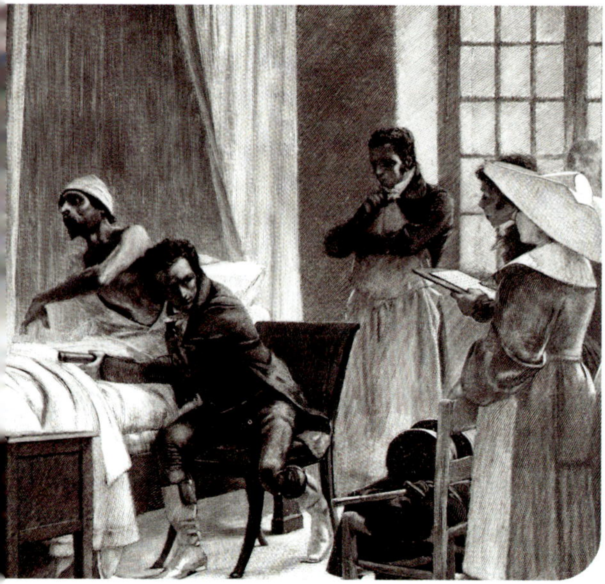

René Laënnec, inventor of the stethoscope, listens to the internal organs of a patient in the early 19th century.

Seeing Inside the Body

Auscultation (listening to breathing and heart sounds through the chest cavity) is a diagnostic method that dates back to ancient Greek times. Today, the familiar tubular rubber device with cup and earpieces is called the stethoscope. The first use of a stethoscope is believed to have been by French physician René Laënnec (1781–1826) in 1816. He was asked to examine a woman with symptoms of heart problems. Rather than press his ear directly against her chest, Laënnec rolled a sheaf of paper into a cylinder and listened to her heart sounds through this. He reported that the sounds could be heard more clearly this way. He soon replaced the paper model with a wooden device. In 1852, American physician George P. Cammann (1804–1863) improved on the basic design by adding tubes and earpieces, one leading to each ear.

In November 1895, German-born Dutch physicist Wilhelm Röntgen (1845–1923) discovered X rays—highly penetrating electromagnetic radiation. By 1898 the British Army was using a mobile X-ray unit in Sudan to locate bone fractures in injured soldiers. However, it was not realized at the time that X rays could be dangerous, and the amount of radiation used for scanning was not reduced until much later.

Since then scientists have developed many new, safer scanning technologies. Ultrasound scans use very high-pitched sound waves, which echo off internal body structures. The first ultrasound images from inside the body were produced by American physician Robert Lee Wild in 1952. A few years later British physician Ian Donald (1910–1987) used ultrasound to see an unborn child in the uterus of a pregnant woman.

In 1972, American physicist Allan MacLeod Cormack (1924–1998) and Godfrey Newbold Hounsfield (1919–2004), a British computer

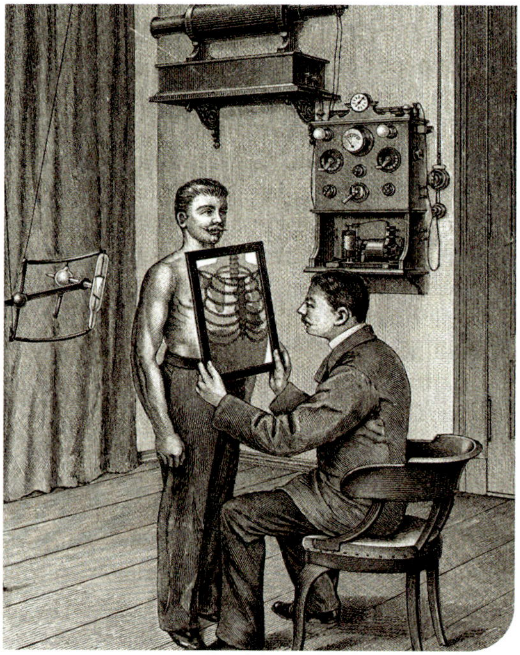

A doctor uses an early X-ray device to look inside a patient's chest. X rays are shining from behind the patient, through the body, and show up on the light-sensitive plate.

ULTRASOUND

Sound waves that have a higher frequency than the sounds humans can hear are ultrasound waves. Ultrasound waves are reflected by small objects, forming echoes that can be used to create images of internal organs. In an ultrasound machine the transducer is often a hand-held device that is passed over the outside of the body (for example, the abdomen of a pregnant woman) to scan the inside; a layer of gel on the skin eases the transmission of waves. The transducer converts electrical energy into ultrasonic waves. Returning echoes are converted into electrical pulses by the transducer. A computer interprets the data and, according to the intensity of the pulses and direction of echoes, produces an image of the scanned object–the unborn baby in the case of a pregnant woman.

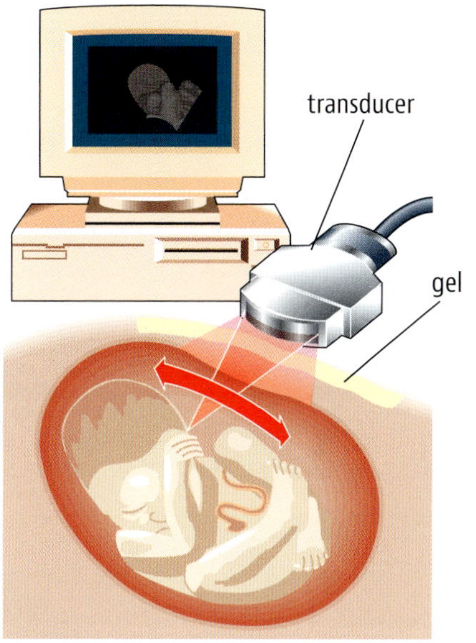

X RAYS AND COMPUTED TOMOGRAPHY

X rays are a type of electromagnetic radiation. Because X rays darken photographic film and can penetrate places that light cannot reach, they can be used to produce images of bones, organs, and internal tissues. An X-ray machine produces X rays by striking a tungsten target with a beam of high-speed electrons. The beam of X rays is passed through the patient's body and picked up by an electronic sensor (similar to the one in a digital or phone camera). Bones absorb a large amount of the X rays, showing up as white "shadows" on the film. Other tissues absorb fewer X rays so show up as gray areas. Computed tomography (CT) involves taking a series of X-ray pictures of cross sections, or slices, through the body. Electronic sensors detect the passage of X rays, sending the data to a computer. The computer combines the X-rayed images to produce a three-dimensional image of the organ scanned.

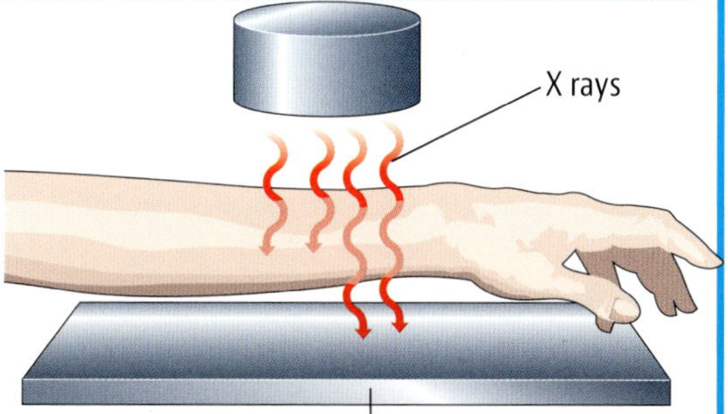

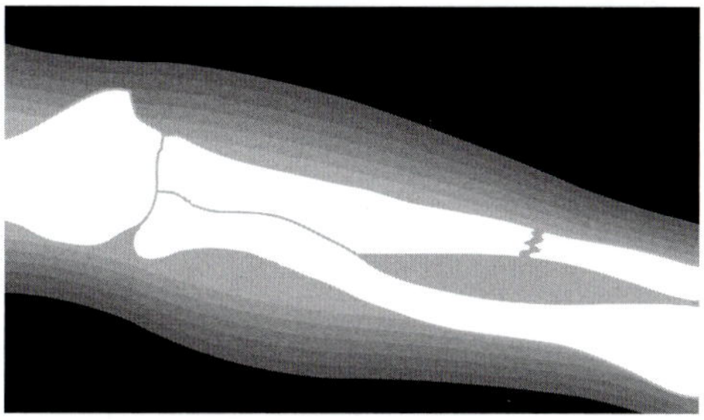

image on X-ray film

MAGNETIC RESONANCE IMAGING

Magnetic resonance imaging (MRI) depends on the tendency of hydrogen atoms to resonate (wobble) and give off radio waves when they are placed in a strong magnetic field. The patient lies on a platform inside what is basically a large, hollow magnet. The angle of the platform can be adjusted to target particular areas of the body. A magnetic field is applied to the body, and this causes the protons of the body's hydrogen atoms to align themselves in the same direction like tiny magnets (normally they point in random directions).

When the MRI machine emits a beam of radio waves, the protons are briefly knocked out of alignment. As they realign themselves, the protons emit faint radio signals that are picked up by the machine's radio-wave receiver. A computer analyzes this data and, according to the length and strength of the detected signals, creates a cross-sectional image of the tissues scanned. MRI can "see through" bones and organs, providing detailed images of, for example, tumors, joints, blood vessels, and the gray matter and white matter in the brain.

A patient lies on a platform inside an MRI scanner. A scan usually takes around 15 to 90 minutes, and the patient must stay completely still during this time..

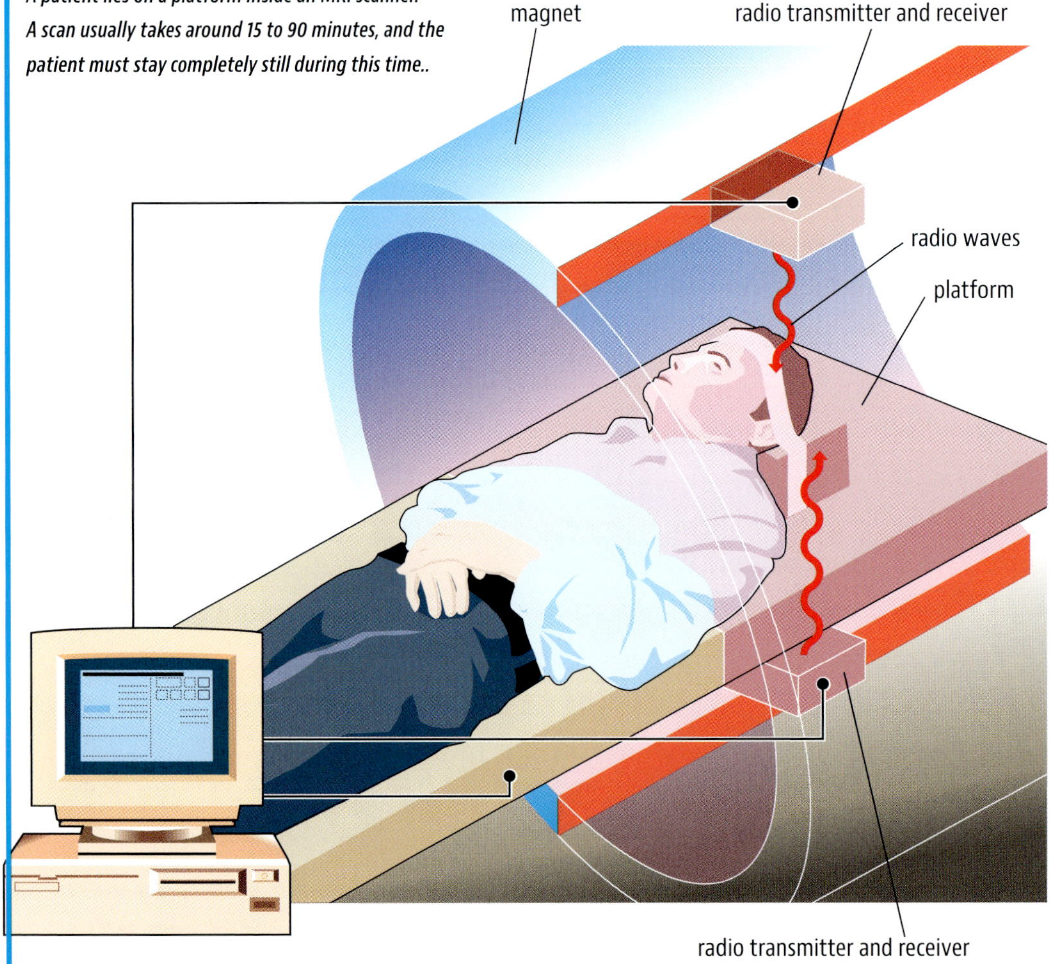

expert and engineer, combined X-ray and computer technology. The technique they developed is called computerized tomography (CT). This method is 100 times more sensitive than traditional X-ray technology and can detect small tumors and blood clots. CT paved the way for other scanning methods, such as positron emission tomography (PET). This technique can track brain activity from second to second and is extremely important for researching mental illness and also for pinpointing brain tumors.

MRI Scanning

In 1977, an American physician, Raymond Damadian (1936–2022), took the first picture inside the human body using a technique called magnetic resonance imaging (MRI). MRI does not involve X rays or radioactive substances and so is a particularly safe method. It is effective in producing an image of the damage to soft tissues such as muscles and nerves and, like PET, gives information about the biological activity of the tissues. Unfortunately, modern scanning methods are expensive and tend to be performed in hospitals and large clinics. In poorer countries, scanners are much less common and doctors use less expensive forms of testing instead.

THREE-STEPS

- The first step in a diagnosis is listening to the patient's account of the illness and checking the medical history of the patient's family.
- After making a physical examination of the patient, the doctor will have in mind a short list of possible diseases.
- Samples of tissue, blood, or urine can then be taken and sent for laboratory testing to confirm the diagnosis.

POSITRON EMISSION TOMOGRAPHY

Positron emission tomography (PET) involves placing part of the patient's body (the head, for example) inside a ring of sensors. The patient is injected with a mildly radioactive substance that gives off positrons (positively charged electrons). The radioactive substance collects in biologically active parts of the body, such as the brain. As the positrons collide with electrons in the brain tissue, they emit gamma rays—a type of short-wave electromagnetic radiation. The sensors detect the points where these rays emerge, and a computer analyzes the data, producing images of slices of the brain that can be made into a three-dimensional image. PET scanners give information about function as well as structure—they can show, for example, which parts of the brain are active when a person is working, listening, reading, or sleeping. PET scans are often used to detect tumors and to examine how the brain functions within mentally ill people.

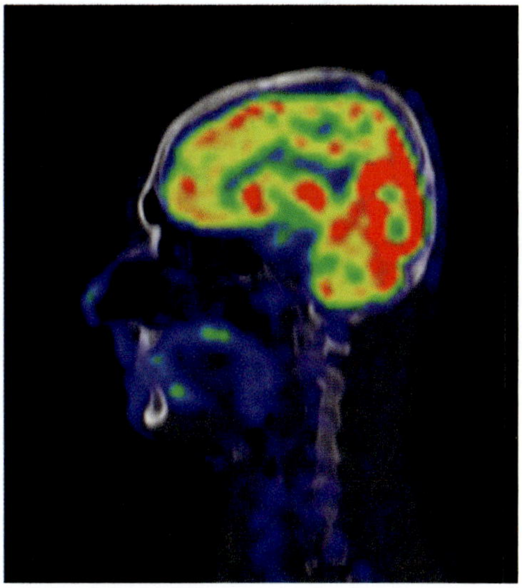

PET scans show up which parts of the brain are active at any given moment, meaning doctors can see the sections controlling different parts of the body.

MODERN SURGERY

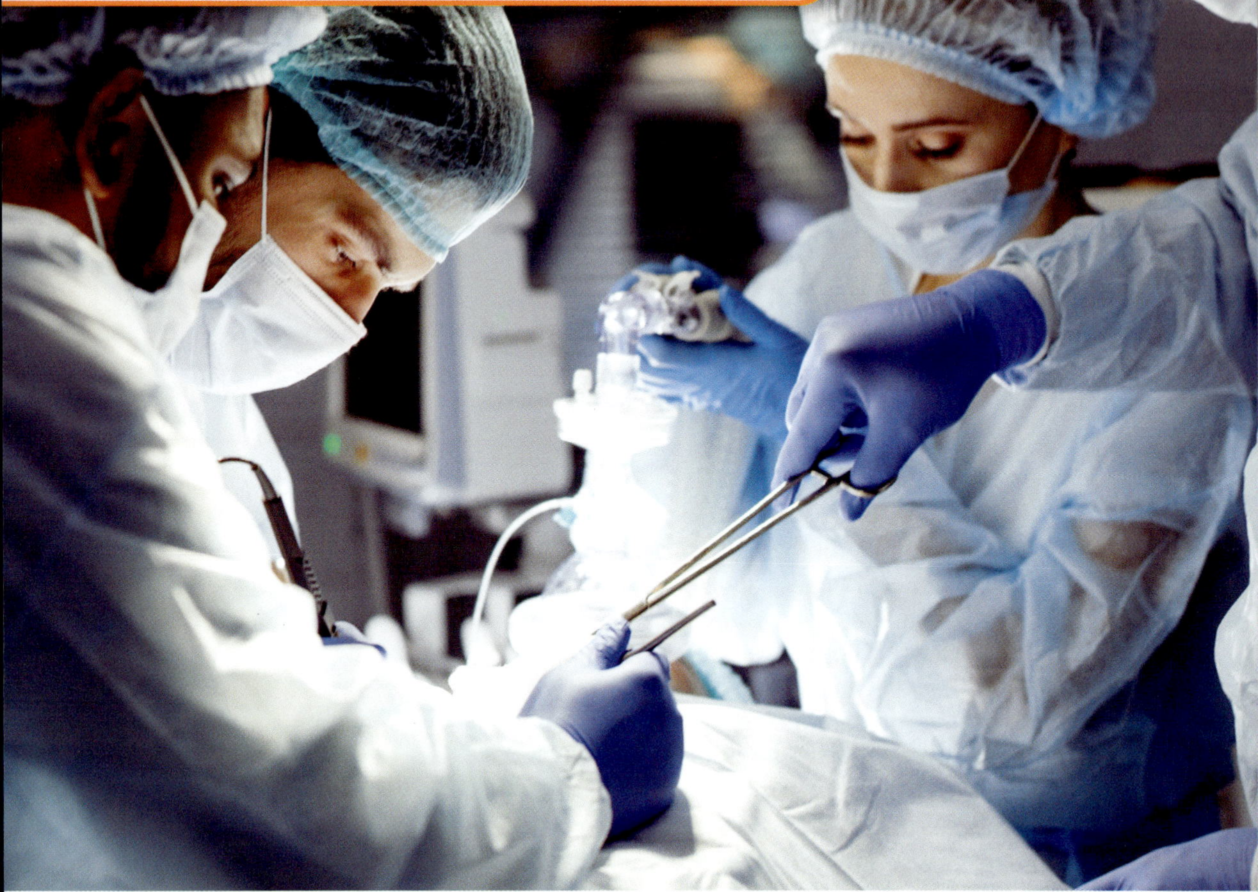

Surgeons do not work alone. Nurses and other doctors assist the lead surgeon and help to keep the patient comfortable.

Medical practitioners have carried out surgical operations since ancient times. The first recorded surgical operation took place 7,000 years ago. However, even today—with modern antiseptics and anesthetics—surgery is still not completely without risk.

Early surgery involved cutting off body parts and sewing up wounded people. Doctors did not often cut deep into a person's body, as patients would nearly always bleed to death during the operation. One of the first successful internal operations was to remove a cancerous part of the stomach. It was carried out by Viennese surgeon Theodor Billroth (1829–1894) in the mid-1800s, and his classic book *General Surgical Pathology and Surgery* (1863) established him as the founder of modern abdominal surgery. Today, Billroth's pioneering operation is still one of the standard treatments for stomach disorders.

During the 20th century many surgical discoveries allowed doctors to develop ways of transplanting organs and giving blood transfusions. Artificial organs and life-support systems have also revolutionized medicine and saved countless lives.

The Age of Machines

Even before immunosuppressant drugs were developed to prevent rejection of transplanted items, doctors were desperately trying to find a way to transplant organs successfully. They were helped by the development of machines that could take over the job of the damaged organ until a donor could be found. In 1914, a team at Johns Hopkins in Baltimore invented the first artificial kidney, or dialysis, machine, which

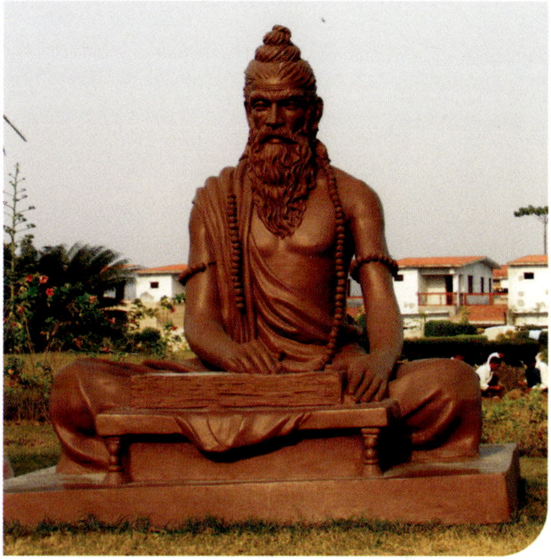

Sushruta, an Indian doctor from around 2,800 years ago, developed many surgical tools. He performed eye surgery to cure blindness and carried out plastic surgery on noses.

TISSUE REJECTION

In 1628, English scientist William Harvey (1578–1657) discovered that the body contained a fixed volume of blood. If a patient lost too much blood, he or she would die, so doctors used a transfusion—replacing it with the blood from another person. However, patients often suffered terrible reactions to the new blood. In 1900, American scientist Karl Landsteiner (1868–1943) discovered this happened because of blood types. A patient could only receive blood of the same type as their own—any another type would cause the blood to form dangerous clots.

The immune system also attacks—or rejects—a transplanted organ. The organ is covered in protein markers called antigens, which show that it comes from outside the body. The first drug to prevent the rejection of transplanted tissues was cortisone. This was used in 1951 to prolong the life of a skin transplant. In 1958, irradiation was used in the first successful kidney transplant between nonidentical twins. Irradiation kills the body's white blood cells, which make up the body's immune system and attack transplanted organs. The main anti-rejection drug used today is cyclosporin. The amazing properties of this drug were discovered by Belgian scientists J.F. Borel in a type of mushroom in 1972.

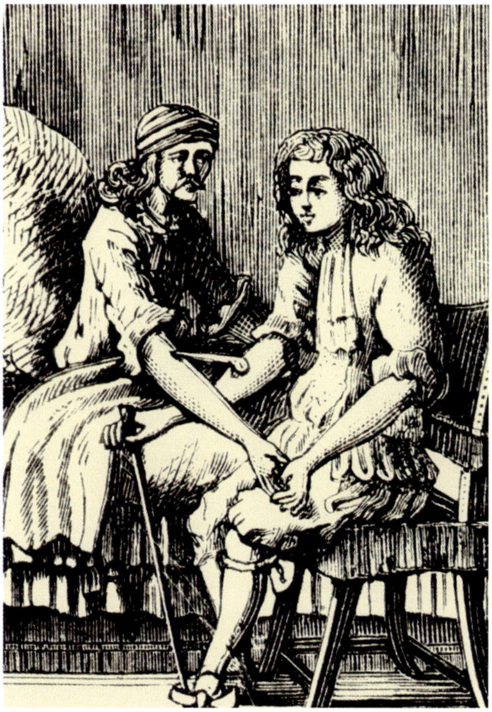

A 17th-century doctor transfuses a patient with his own blood through a tube connecting the blood vessels in their arms.

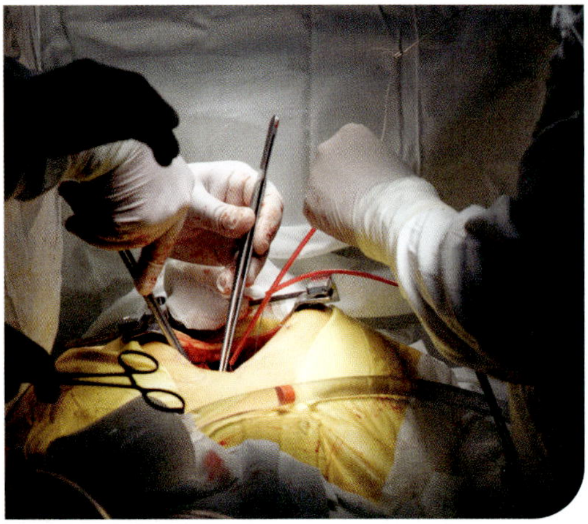

they tested on dogs with kidney disease. However, these experiments were forgotten by everyone except a physician in the Netherlands called Willem Kolff (1911–2009). In 1943, Kolff invented a kidney dialysis machine for humans, using sausage casing for the tubes. The first kidney transplant in which the patient survived was carried out in 1950 by doctor Richard H. Lawler (1895–1982).

Surgeons operating on a heart. The problems of stopping and restarting blood flow between the heart, lungs, and the rest of the body during operations were solved in the late 20th century.

ABO BLOOD GROUPS AND TRANSFUSIONS

There are four blood groups: A, B, AB, and O. If a person with blood group A received blood of type B during a transfusion, the result would be fatal. People with blood group A produce anti-B antibodies, which "attack" antigen B (found on type B blood cells), making the blood clot. People with blood group AB produce neither anti-A nor anti-B antibodies, so they can receive blood of type A, B, AB, or O. People with blood group O, however, produce both anti-A and anti-B antibodies, so they can only receive type O blood. In practice, matching blood types are given whenever possible, and there are other blood grouping systems—the Rhesus system, for example—that have to be considered as well as the standard ABO system.

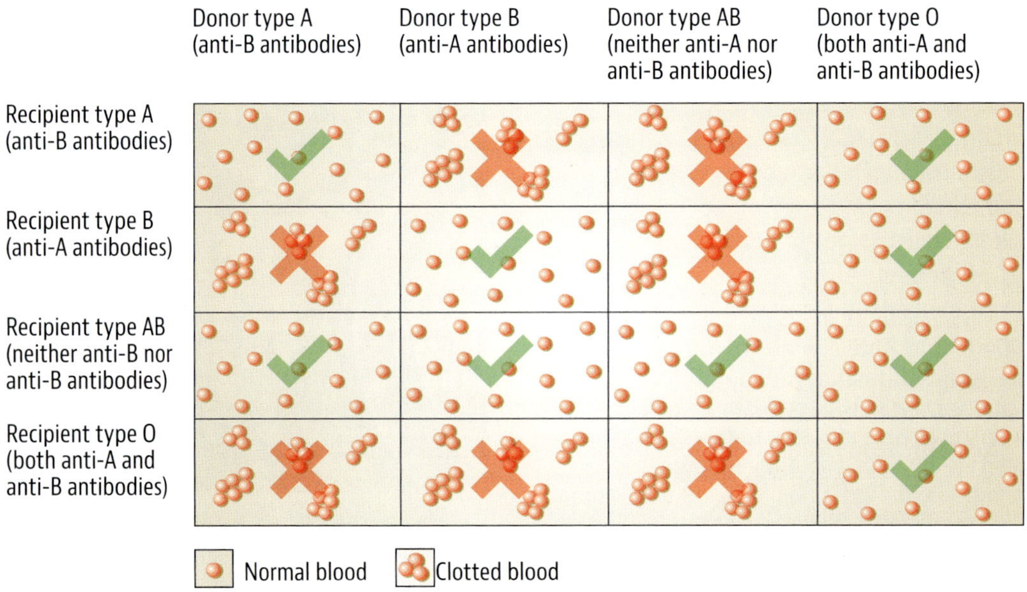

Transplanting a heart was much more difficult. A heart must be removed and transplanted within a few hours. There is also the problem of keeping the blood moving around the body while the surgery is being performed. In 1930, American surgeon John H. Gibbon (1903–1973) developed a heart-lung machine that would pump oxygen into the patient's blood during heart surgery. In 1954, Gibbon used this machine to operate on a 19-year-old girl. The machine kept her alive for 27 minutes during the operation. In 1961, American surgeon Norman Shumway (1923–2006) invented a machine that kept the patient's blood flowing after surgery until the new heart was ready to take over. This machine allowed the first human-to-human heart operation to be carried out in 1967, by South African surgeon Christiaan Barnard (1922–2001).

DIALYSIS MACHINE

Dialysis machines have to perform the jobs that kidneys normally do: they must filter the blood of waste products and remove excess fluid from the body, which is then sent to the bladder and eventually excreted as liquid urine.

1 Blood is taken from the patient and pumped to the dialysis machine.
2 The dialysis machine contains a fluid called dialysate, which consists of water, salts, and other solutions.
3 Inside the dialysis machine a membrane with tiny holes in it separates the blood from the dialysate. Wastes and excess fluid pass from the blood into the dialysate, which carries them away.
4 The cleansed blood is then returned to the patient.

Dialysis can be performed at out-patient clinics, but it can also be done at home by the patients themselves. In another type of dialysis, pioneered in the 1970s, patients are simply attached to a bag of dialysate, and a membrane inside the body is used to filter the blood, which does not need to be pumped out of the body.

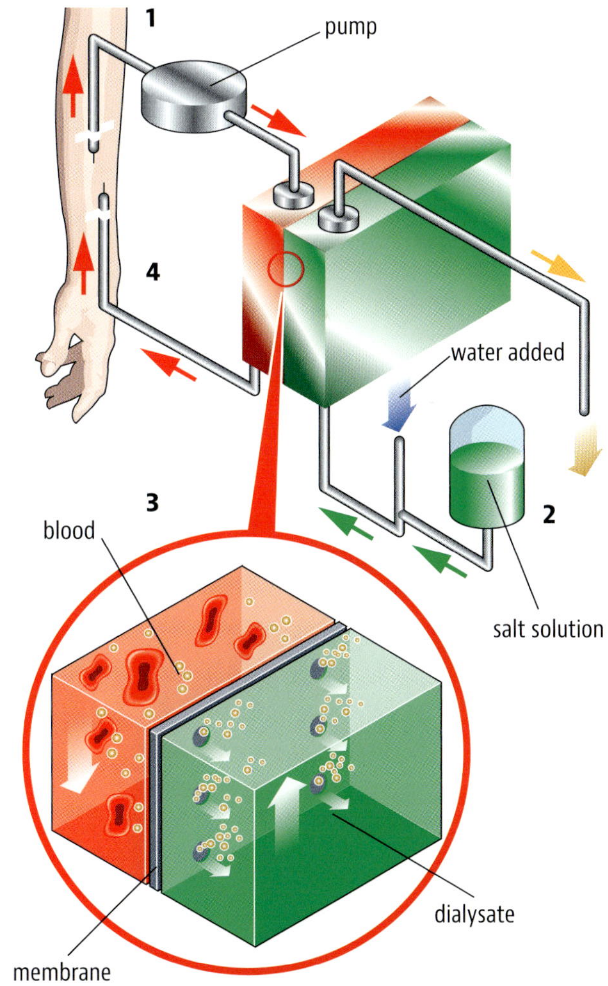

In addition to heart surgery, the 20th century has seen the development of new ways to keep a damaged heart working. For example, pacemakers were invented in the 1950s, and in 1951 the first workable synthetic heart valve was designed and inserted into a patient by Charles Antony Hufnagel (1916–1989). In 1968, René Favaloro carried out the first coronary bypass operation. The coronary artery carries the main blood supply of the heart and can be blocked by fatty deposits—the bypass involved taking the damaged piece of artery away and replacing it with a vein cut from the patient's leg.

Artificial Body Parts

Sometimes, however, even surgery cannot solve a serious heart problem. Willem Kolff began research into developing a total replacement heart in the 1950s, and in 1957

HEART-LUNG MACHINE

Heart-lung machines temporarily take over the functions of the heart and lungs, allowing surgeons to carry out otherwise impossible operations in the chest. An oxygenator performs the task of the lungs—adding the vital gas oxygen to blood, which is then pumped around the body by a pump functioning as the heart. Oxygen is needed for body cells to work. The use of a heart-lung machine is limited to a few hours, since it reduces the blood supply to vital organs.

1 Blood is taken from the main veins that bring blood to the heart.
2 This blood is oxygen-poor, and it is delivered to the artificial lung (oxygenator), where it picks up much more oxygen.
3 This oxygen-rich blood is pumped through a temperature controller and a filter (to prevent clots forming) before it is passed back to a main artery, from where it circulates around the body.
4 Blood leaving the heart is channeled through a defoamer (to remove bubbles) and sent to the oxygenator.

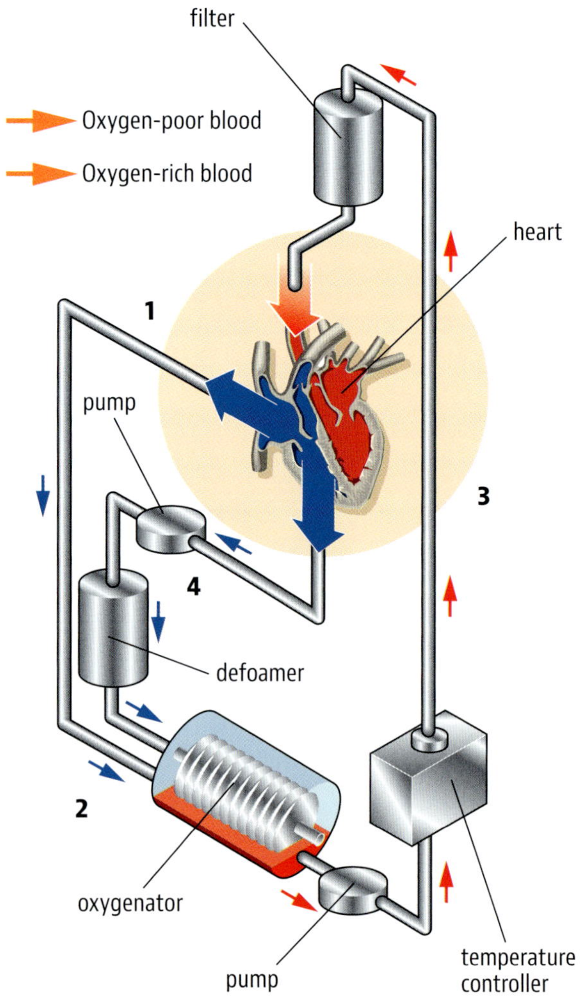

he implanted his first model into a dog. The dog survived for 90 minutes. In 1970, Robert Jarvik devised an artificial heart made of polyurethane (a type of plastic) and fiber glass. This was first used in a human in 1982. The patient survived for 112 days. The longest time a patient survived was 20 months.

The most commonly used artificial body replacement is the hip. Hip replacements became possible with the development of plastics and acrylics before WWII (1939–1945), but there were problems with artificial hips until 1960, when British surgeon John Charnley (1911–1982) developed a hip joint that used

PACEMAKERS

The heart has its own electrical system, called a pacemaker, which acts to keep it beating regularly. Artificial pacemakers are implanted in the chest to send electrical impulses to the heart when its own pacemaker is not working. The first of these devices was made in 1958 and implanted by Swedish doctor Ake Sening in 1960. Early models had a power source under the skin and used mercury-zinc batteries that ran out after two or three years. In 1973, a lithium-iodide power cell was developed that lasts more than six years. Modern devices all use this kind of battery.

Internal pacemakers are implanted in the chest. An insulated electrical wire is inserted into the heart via a vein. A fixing mechanism such as a staple holds the electrode in place, next to the part of the heart needing stimulation. The other end of the wire plugs into the pacemaker. Electrical impulses stimulate the heart to beat. Some pacemakers discharge electrical impulses at a fixed rate; others only discharge impulses when they identify that the heart has slowed down or a beat is missed.

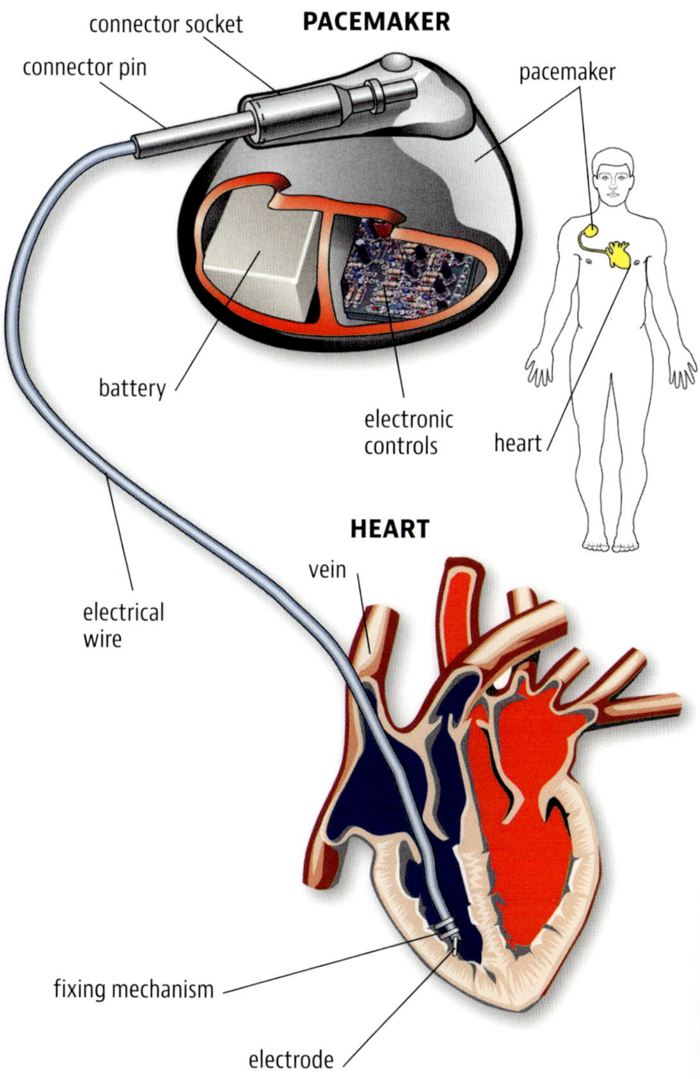

two different materials: the head of the femur (the long leg bone) was replaced with a stainless steel ball, and the ball of the hip joint was lined with a slippery plastic called Teflon. This allowed the steel ball to move around more freely.

Keyhole Surgery

If surgeons do not have to make large cuts to perform surgery, the patient recovers much faster. A minimally invasive surgery was developed in the 1980s using tools known as endoscopes. These tools are equipped with lasers instead of scalpels. Endoscopes can be inserted into the body through openings such as the mouth, or they can be inserted through small incisions in a procedure called "keyhole" surgery. Extra tubes in the endoscope suck out blood or pump in replacement fluids to flush an organ clean. Keyhole surgeons can even inflate small balloons inside arteries to push out fatty deposits.

SITES OF POSSIBLE IMPLANTS

Implants are natural and artificial materials inserted into the body for medical purposes. Many implants repair or replace a part of the body that no longer works properly. The lens in an eye, for example, or even the whole eyeball, can be replaced. Pacemakers keep the heart beating regularly, and diseased heart valves can be replaced with flexible plastic ones. Hip, knee, elbow, shoulder, and finger joints can be replaced with artificial substitutes, made from metal, plastic, or ceramic. Artificial blood vessels made from synthetic materials can replace diseased sections of arteries.

Implants containing radioactive materials can be inserted into tissue to treat cancers, and others containing drugs (such as contraceptives or pain killers) are inserted to release the drug slowly over a long period of time. Some implants, such as silicone breast implants, are used to change a person's appearance.

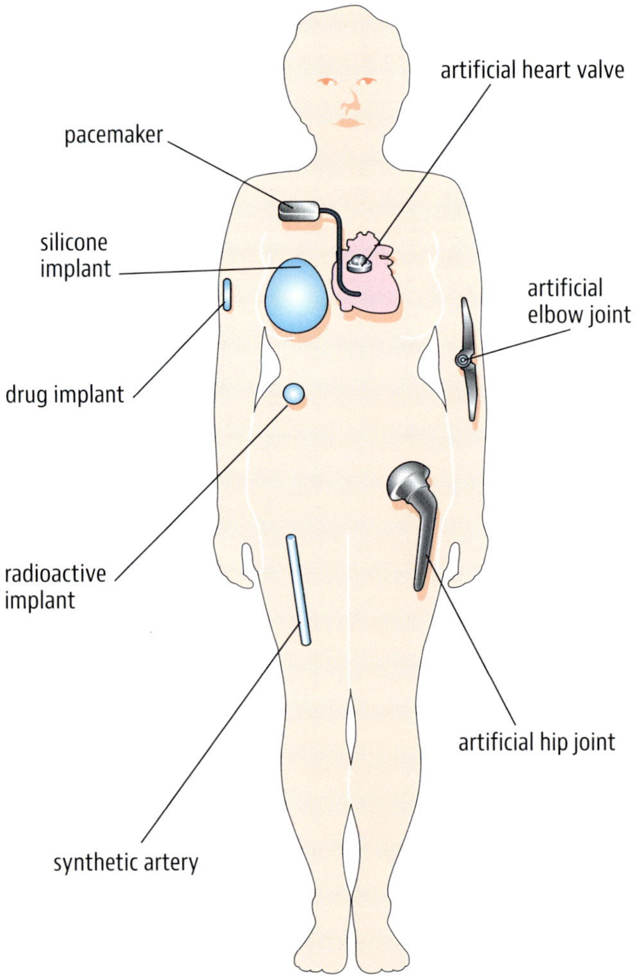

HEARING AIDS

Many people with normal hearing may think that people who are deaf cannot hear anything at all. This is generally not the case. A complete inability to hear, or profound deafness, affects a small minority of deaf people. Most have conductive or sensori-neural hearing loss. Both of these disorders allow at least some types of sound, especially deep, booming vibrations, to be heard.

Conductive hearing loss is caused by sound being unable to pass normally from the outer to the inner ear. This may be the result of blockage or damage to the middle ear. Conductive hearing loss causes all sounds to be heard much more quietly. Loud voices will sound like whispers, while soft voices may not be heard at all. Sensori-neural hearing loss is the result of damage to the inner ear and causes sounds to become distorted. It is less common than conductive hearing loss, but more likely to be permanent. In most cases of sensori-neural hearing loss, high-frequency sounds are cut out. The result is that the long, rounded vowels in speech are audible but most clicking consonant sounds are not.

Hearing aids can help most people with moderate hearing loss. The simplest devices fit in or behind the ear and work like miniature amplifiers, making quiet sounds louder to cancel out the effect of conductive hearing loss. People with sensori-neural hearing loss often use digital hearing aids, which can be tuned to boost the specific sound frequencies they no longer hear. People with severe hearing loss who can't use a normal hearing aid may benefit from a cochlear implant (pictured below). This device is surgically implanted into the inner ear. A microphone unit fitted behind the outer ear converts sounds into a simplified sound signal, which is transmitted into the head, bypassing the middle ear.

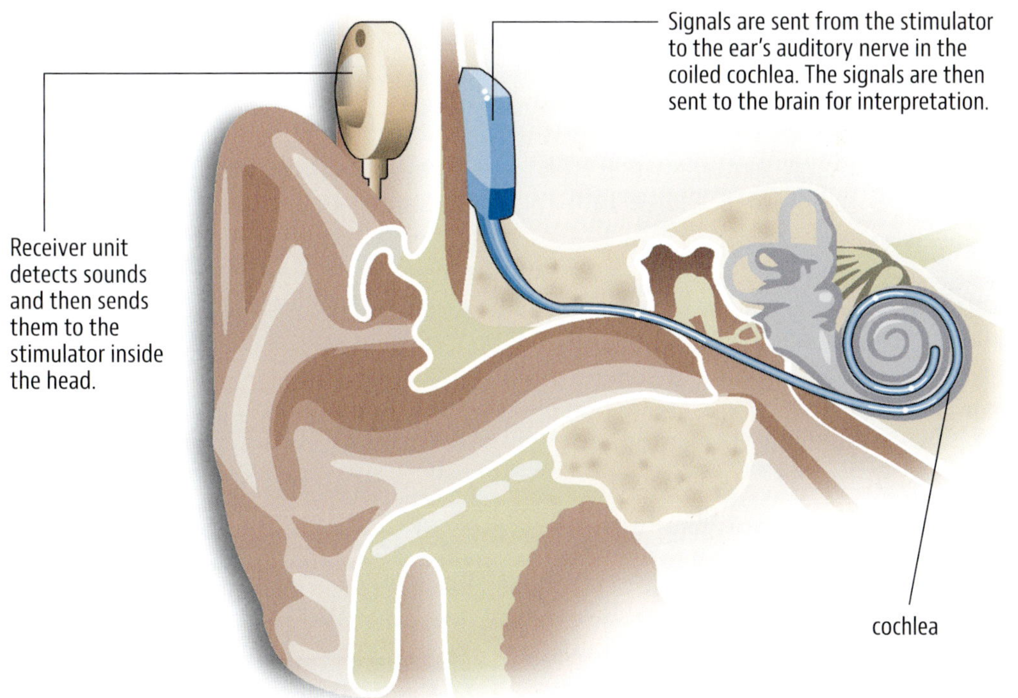

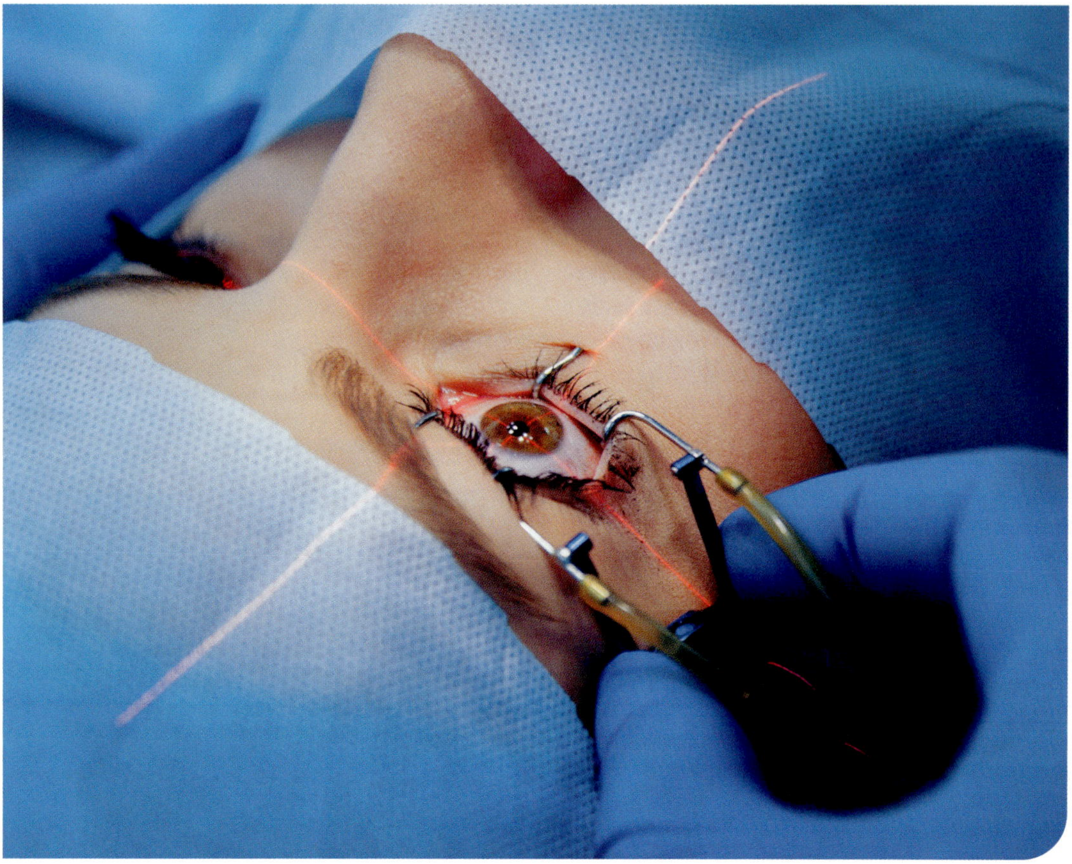

Myopia, or short-sightedness, can sometimes be cured by cutting the cornea (eye covering) with a laser. The cuts are placed precisely so they help to focus light into the eye correctly.

Lasers and shock waves allow some medical conditions to be treated without the need for surgery at all. In 1982, surgeons developed a machine that can destroy kidney stones using powerful shock waves. The stones, which before this invention had to be removed by surgery, are broken down into tiny grains, which pass out through the patient's urine. In 1986, German scientist Ludwig Demling used a laser attached to an endoscope to treat gallstones. He inserted the endoscope into the gallbladder and fired laser shots at the stones to destroy them without damaging the surrounding tissue.

Cryosurgery (using extremely low temperatures to destroy dead, damaged, or cancerous tissue) has also revolutionized surgery. Irving Coope first used liquid nitrogen in cryosurgery in 1960. This type of surgery is painless, and there is no risk of bleeding.

FACTS AND FIGURES

- More than 4,000 heart transplant operations are carried out in the United States each year.
- The first patient to receive a heart transplant, Louis Washkansky in South Africa in 1967, died after 18 days.
- Full recovery from a heart transplant can take around three months.

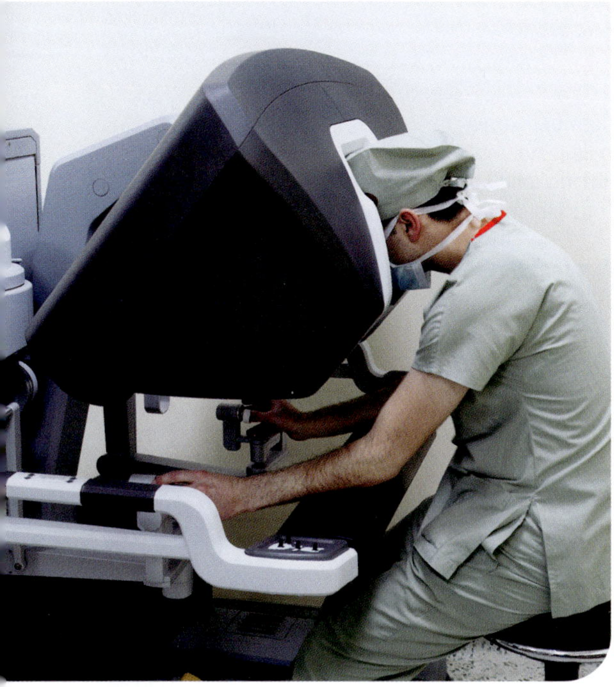

A surgeon operates using a robot. The doctor views the patient in virtual reality, while the robot makes precise cuts.

Noninvasive surgical techniques, such as the use of lasers and endoscopes, have cut down drastically the amount of time needed for the surgery itself and for the patients' recovery afterward. This has led to the development of surgery on an outpatient basis, with hospital admittance, surgical operation, and discharge all sometimes occurring in just one day. As a result, most routine procedures, such as removal of the appendix or tonsils, can be performed safely with a minimum of distress to the patient.

Stem cell therapy has been used to treat some conditions where once surgeons would have operated. This includes dealing with athritic joints. Stem cells also have much wider applications, which include healing wounds and dealing with fertility issues. However, the creation of large numbers of stem cells is an extremely controversial area of science.

SOCIETY AND INVENTIONS

Cosmetic Plastic Surgery

Plastic surgery is any operation that reshapes or reconstructs the body. Reconstructive surgery has a long history treating, for example, disfiguring burns and congenital (in-born) disorders such as severe cleft palates, in which the top lip is actually connected to the nostrils.

Many of the techniques of modern plastic surgery originate with surgeons who were repairing the wounds and disfigurements of soldiers. Today, doctors can change the shape of a person's jaw, nose, ears, breasts, and many other body parts, and they can remove excess fat, smooth out wrinkles (below), and transplant hair. But people's expectations of cosmetic surgery are often too great. It cannot produce a dramatic change in personality or stop the depression that a person may blame on their appearance.

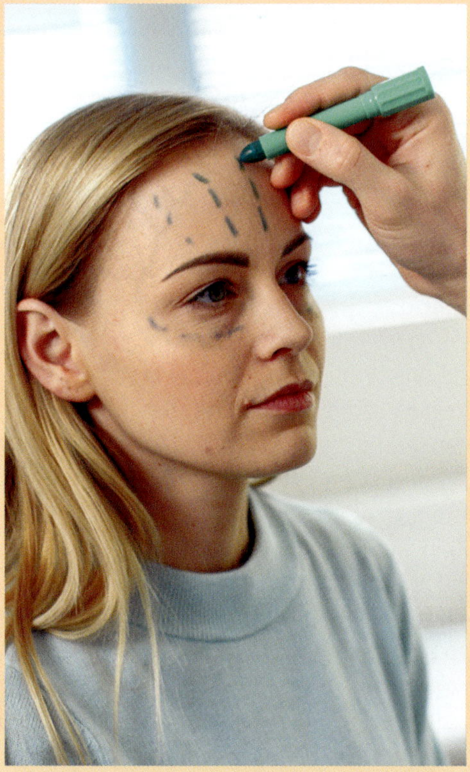

REPRODUCTION AND GENETICS

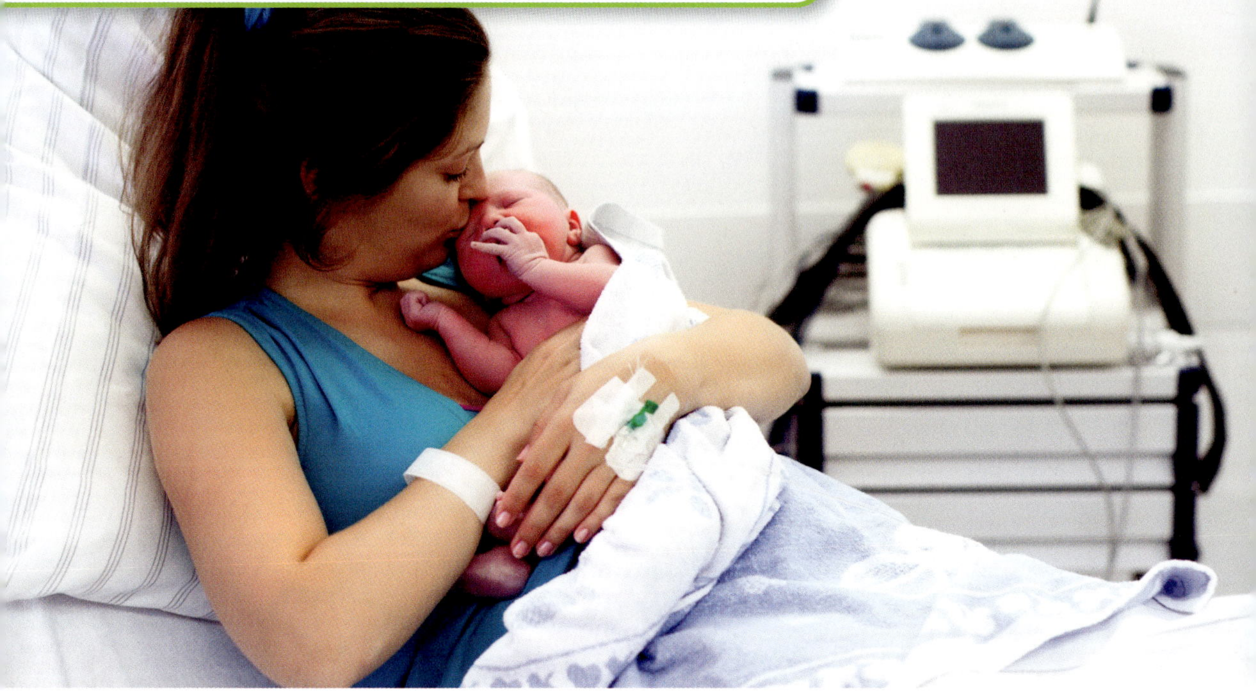

In wealthy countries most babies are born in hospital, where doctors are on hand to help if problems occur.

For centuries, men dominated medicine. However, women practitioners play equally important roles in medical practice today, with obstetrics, the medicine of pregnancy and birth, being just one specialism.

In ancient Greece and Rome most doctors were men. The few women who practiced medicine tended to specialize in female ailments, cared for pregnant women, and attended births. However, the best-known ancient text on gynecology (the female reproductive system) was written by a man, Soranus of Ephesus, a Greek physician who lived around 100 CE.

In the United States and Europe during the 18th and 19th centuries midwives were mostly women. However, as medicine became more scientific and technological, and more equipment was used, male doctors began to take a greater interest in taking control of the childbirth process. In many cultures this trend has continued right up to the present day. Many women now give birth in the hospital under the supervision of a doctor, although many women have their babies at home with planned home births.

In the 1920s, childbirth was still a hazardous event. In this period in the United States at least 17 percent of mothers died during childbirth. Authorities identified several factors as responsible for the high death rate, ranging from poor hygiene and housing to lack of professional care before, during, and after birth. Prenatal (before-birth) care for the mother and unborn child was introduced on a wide scale.

New techniques to monitor the health of the unborn baby (fetus) were, however, slow to emerge. In the 19th century French obstetrician Adolphe Pinard designed a stethoscope to detect fetal heartbeats. He also introduced a massage technique for turning the baby into the correct head-down position for birth. In 1916, Norwegian obstetrician Christian Kielland introduced a new design of forceps for gripping the baby's head accurately to assist during difficult births. Despite their effectiveness many doctors used forceps without adequate training, and in some cases they made injury to the mother or baby more likely. In the 1930s the increasing use of blood transfusions helped save lives, as did the introduction of antibacterial drugs called sulfonamides.

For mothers giving birth in the hospital drugs such as morphine and scopolamine were injected to ease pain. The trend toward increasing technological control of childbirth continued between the 1930s and 1980s. Better forms of painkiller were developed, and epidural anesthesia (in which anesthetic is injected into the lower back, numbing all sensation below that point) allowed mothers to stay awake during caesarean sections. This is when the baby is delivered surgically through the mother's abdomen in cases where it might be difficult to give birth through the birth canal.

HYGIENE SAVES LIVES

Hungarian physician Ignaz Semmelweis (1818–1865) noticed while working in maternity wards that mothers under the supervision of female midwives had a better chance of surviving childbirth than those who were looked after by male doctors. The doctors often carried out autopsies (dissections of dead bodies to decide the cause of death), and then helped deliver babies—without washing their hands or changing their clothes. When Semmelweis made his medical students wash their hands in disinfectant before dealing with patients, the death rate fell among childbearing women.

This is an example of the use of antisepsis—methods of hygiene that kill germs, or microorganisms such as bacteria and viruses. At the time no one knew these tiny organisms were the cause of diseases, but Semmelweis's approach worked nonetheless. It was not until about 20 years later that French chemist Louis Pasteur (1822–1895) showed a link between microorganisms and disease.

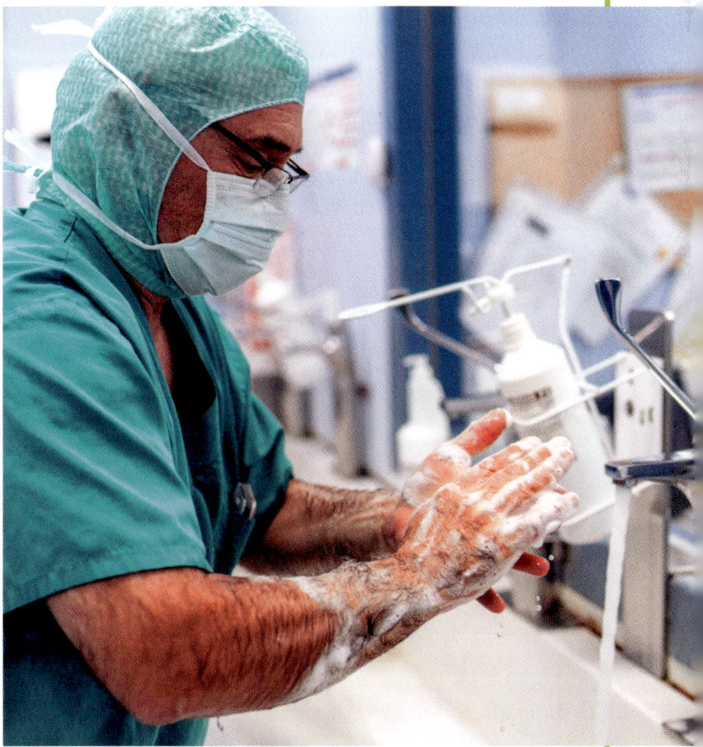

Since the mid-1800s, keeping hands and clothing scrupulously clean has been known to be crucially important in preventing infection when treating patients.

Controlling Fertility

Reducing fertility—the ability to conceive a child—was tried in many civilizations, while contraception, to stop fertilization of an egg by sperm, has been practiced for many centuries. In ancient Egypt over 4,000 years ago women used pessaries (substances placed in the vagina) made from items such as honey and crocodile dung. This method worked to some extent, because the concoctions made the vagina unwelcoming for active sperm. However, the method was far from foolproof, and some of the pessaries were actually dangerous. By the late Middle Ages contraception had taken an even more dangerous turn. Some women took poisonous herbal mixtures to reduce fertility.

Italian biologist Gabriello Fallopius (1523–1562) is credited with inventing the linen condom around 1550. This was designed to prevent transmission of sexually transmitted diseases (STDs) rather than to prevent pregnancy, although it may have worked reasonably well at combating both. With the advent of the human immunodeficiency virus (HIV) in the 1980s, the disease-prevention role of the condom was once again recognized.

German physician Frederick Adolphe Wilde made the first versions of the diaphragm in the 1820s, but in 1882 German doctor W.P.J. Mesinga devised a larger version made from latex rubber, similar to those used today.

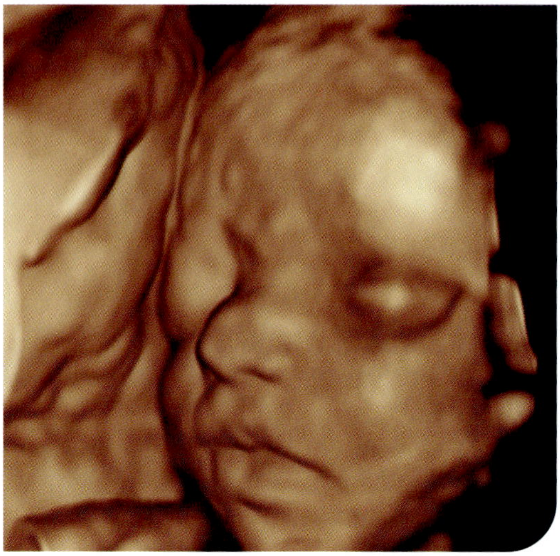

A 3D (three-dimensional) scan of a developing fetus in its mother's womb.

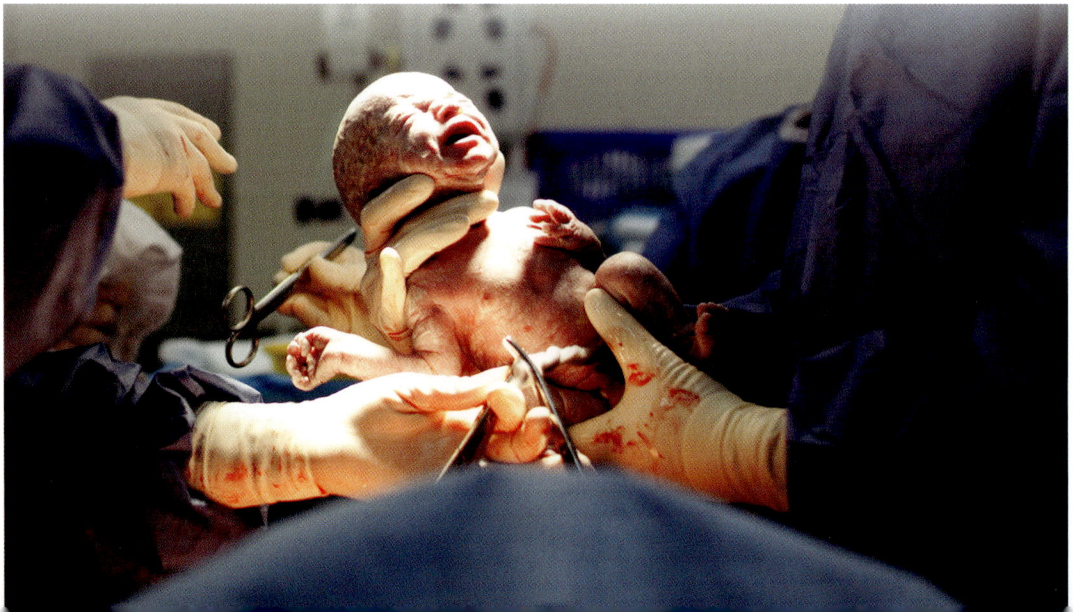

A baby delivered by caesarian section, in which surgeons cut into the womb to extract the baby, for example if the birth canal has become blocked or if the mother is experiencing difficulties..

CHROMOSOMES, DNA, AND GENES

Inside the nucleus of every human body cell are 46 chromosomes. In the male and female sex cells (sperm and eggs) there are only 23 chromosomes—so when a sperm fertilizes an egg, the resulting cell, which develops into an embryo, has its quota of 46 chromosomes. In this way a baby inherits its chromosomes from its parents—half coming from the mother and half from the father.

Each chromosome consists of a strand of coiled up deoxyribonucleic acid (DNA). DNA is like a twisted ladder (the double helix), the rungs of which are made up of four chemicals called bases. A gene is made up of several hundred or several thousand bases on a separated strand of the double helix. The order in which the bases appear dictates which proteins are made. Proteins are the building blocks of cells and determine every feature of a person. One faulty gene can mean a certain protein is not produced, causing a genetic disorder. Genetic disorders include Huntingdon's Disease and cystic fibrosis, which are passed on from a person's parents.

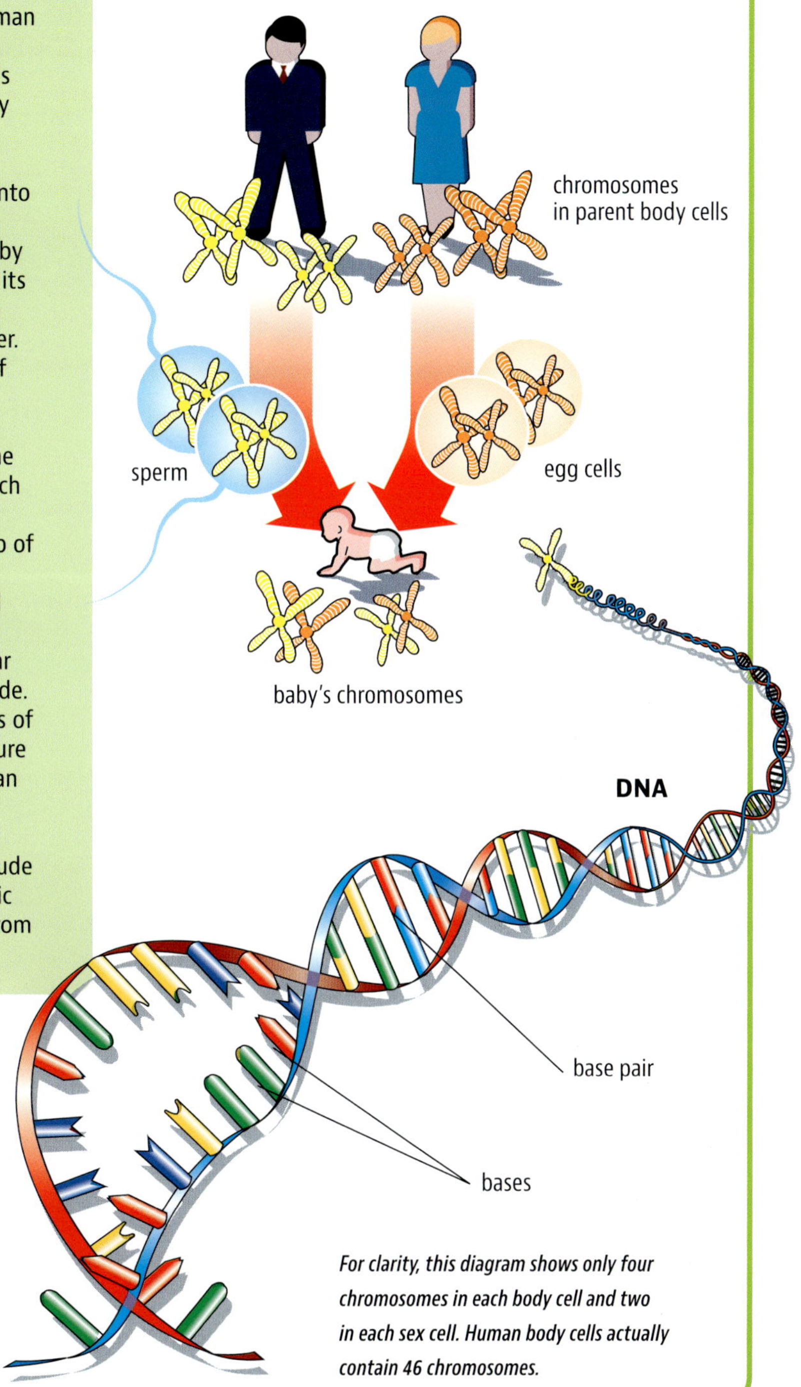

For clarity, this diagram shows only four chromosomes in each body cell and two in each sex cell. Human body cells actually contain 46 chromosomes.

METHODS OF CONTRACEPTION

For a child to be conceived, a female egg has to be fertilized by (fused with) a male sperm. Women store eggs in their ovaries, which release the eggs to travel down the fallopian tubes and into the uterus, where a baby will grow from an egg if it is fertilized. Male produce sperm in their testes, which release the sperm to travel down each vas deferens and out of the penis. During intercourse the male's penis delivers sperm to the woman's vagina, and the sperm can travel past the cervix into the uterus, where an egg can be fertilized.

Contraceptive devices interfere with this process, preventing conception. To prevent sperm entering the uterus, condoms can cover the penis or vagina, and diaphragms and caps are worn by women over the cervix. IUDs (or coils) make the uterus inhospitable for fertilized eggs.

Women can take pills that either interfere with the release of eggs (ovulation), make the cervical mucus (thick, slimy fluid) impenetrable by sperm, or affect the lining of the uterus so that eggs cannot implant. A male Pill has been researched with the aim of preventing sperm being produced. The Pill has the advantage of being reversible: its effects end when a person stops taking it. Sterilization (cutting of each vas deferens in men and the fallopian tubes in women) is the most foolproof contraceptive method but it is often irreversible.

SITES OF ACTION OF CONTRACEPTIVE DEVICES

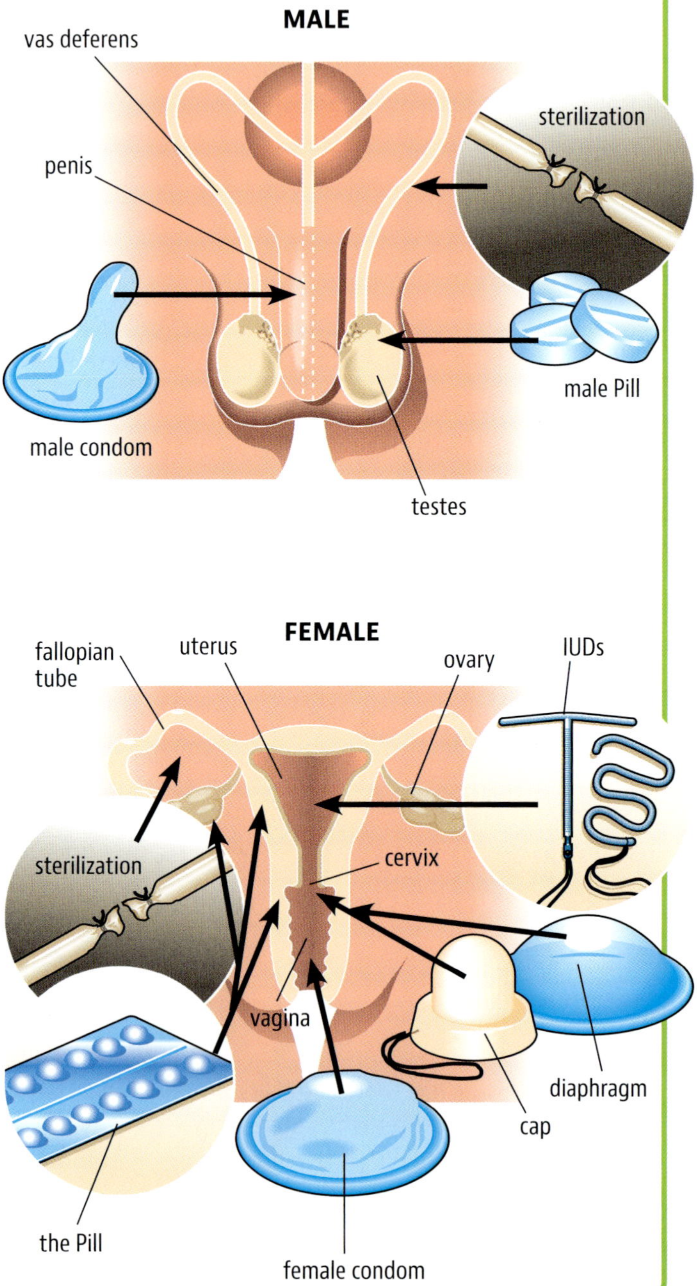

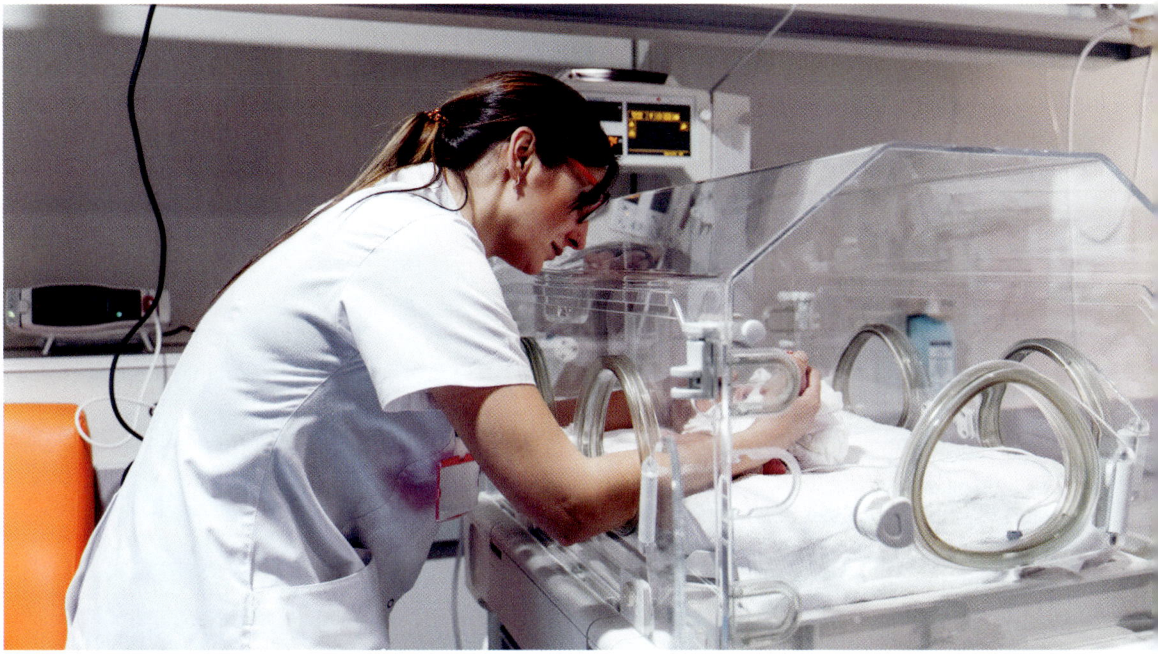

Babies that are born earlier than normal are often kept in a controlled environment called an incubator for a little while. The machine keeps them warm while they complete their development.

The first intrauterine device (IUD), or coil, was a silver spiral designed by German doctor Ernst Grafenberg in 1928. Today, IUDs come in many shapes and sizes, and usually contain plastic and metal. Some are impregnated with the hormone progesterone to prevent the release of eggs.

Perhaps the greatest revolution in contraception came with the advent of the contraceptive pill, sometimes just called "the Pill". In the 1950s, several chemists were involved in its early development. Progesterone—which is produced by women's bodies to prepare the uterus for pregnancy—is the Pill's main ingredient. It prevents a woman ovulating (releasing eggs). Progesterone is present in only tiny quantities in humans and other animals, but during the late 1940s American chemist Russell E. Marker (1902–1984) found a way of converting substances in the wild yam plant into usable progesterone. During the 1950s researchers developed synthetic (artificial) progesterones that were more powerful than the natural form, and which could be swallowed and absorbed by the body. Between 1954 and 1959, the American biologists Gregory Pincus (1903–1967) and John Rock (1890–1984) tested the first contraceptive pill. By the mid-1970s more than 50 million women were using it as birth control.

Fertility Treatment

There are many reasons why couples may not be able to have children. The woman's fallopian tubes may be blocked, or sometimes mucus (thick, slippery fluid) in the cervix kills the man's sperm. Sometimes the man may produce relatively few sperm, or those that he does produce are defective in some way. In the last 50 years many techniques have been developed to try to help people overcome such problems.

In Vitro Fertilization

The most publicized procedure to help fertility is the so-called "test-tube baby" technique, which was developed by British physicians Patrick Steptoe (1913–1988) and Robert Edwards (1925–2013). This method, in which an egg is combined with sperm outside the body, resulted in the first test-tube baby—Louise Brown—being born in July 1978. Despite the name, test tubes are not involved. The scientific name is *in vitro* (Latin for "in glass") fertilization, or IVF. Worldwide, millions of babies have been conceived by IVF, but it is a difficult and costly method.

Genetic Screening

Every cell in every living thing contains genetic (inherited) material called DNA, which

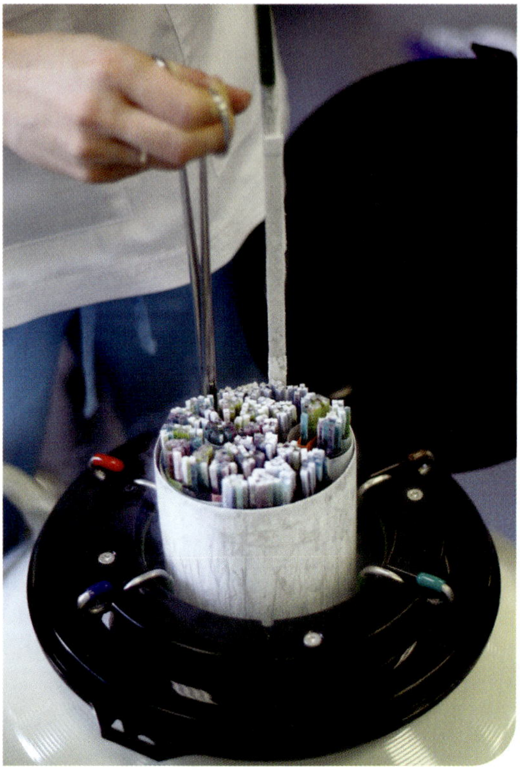

Some of the elements involved in fertility, such as eggs, sperm, and even embyros can be stored in a deep freeze for several years. The freezer uses liquid nitrogen to keep things very cold.

SOCIETY AND INVENTIONS

IVF: Moral Issues

The IVF technique raises many moral and ethical questions. Are the embryos (the clumps of cells that will eventually develop into fetuses) growing in the dish actually human beings, or rather, are they human beings-to-be? If any of them are not implanted in the mother's body, should they be kept for other purposes?

Unused embryos are often frozen so the parents can use them later if they wish to have a baby. With permission, some embryos are also used in experiments, provided they are not allowed to grow beyond 14 days. The controls on experimentation vary greatly from country to country, and such experiments are naturally extremely controversial.

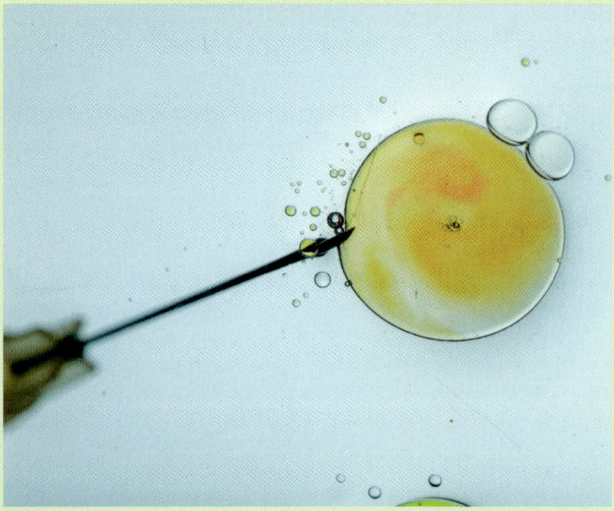

This close-up photograph shows an egg being injected with sperm in a laboratory.

carries the instructions for the development of all characteristics of the organism. For example, whether you are short or tall, have blond or brown hair, and have blue or green eyes is determined by your DNA.

Genetic screening involves examining a person's DNA to check for potential problems. In 1952, the British physician D.C.A. Bevis described the process of amniocentesis, a technique used for sampling the fluid surrounding an unborn baby in which some of the baby's cells are collected so that they can be checked for any genetic abnormalities. The technique is used to test for Down's syndrome, spina bifida, and other genetic conditions. Such screening methods are still important today.

The Human Genome Project

In the 1990s, a research project was launched to decipher the base sequence of every human gene and map the human genome

IVF TREATMENT

1 Early in a woman's menstrual cycle she is injected with fertility drugs so that she produces three or more eggs at one time.
2 The ripening of eggs in the ovaries is monitored by a series of ultrasound scans.
3 Immediately before ovulation (the release of eggs from the ovaries) the most ripe egg cells are removed from one of the ovaries using a fine, hollow needle.
4 The eggs are placed in a glass dish and fertilized with the partner's male sperm.
5 Several fertilized eggs that have begun to grow into embryos (clumps of cells that grow into fetuses) are placed in the mother's uterus. If IVF is successful (success rates are under 50 percent) the mother will probably be carrying more than one child.

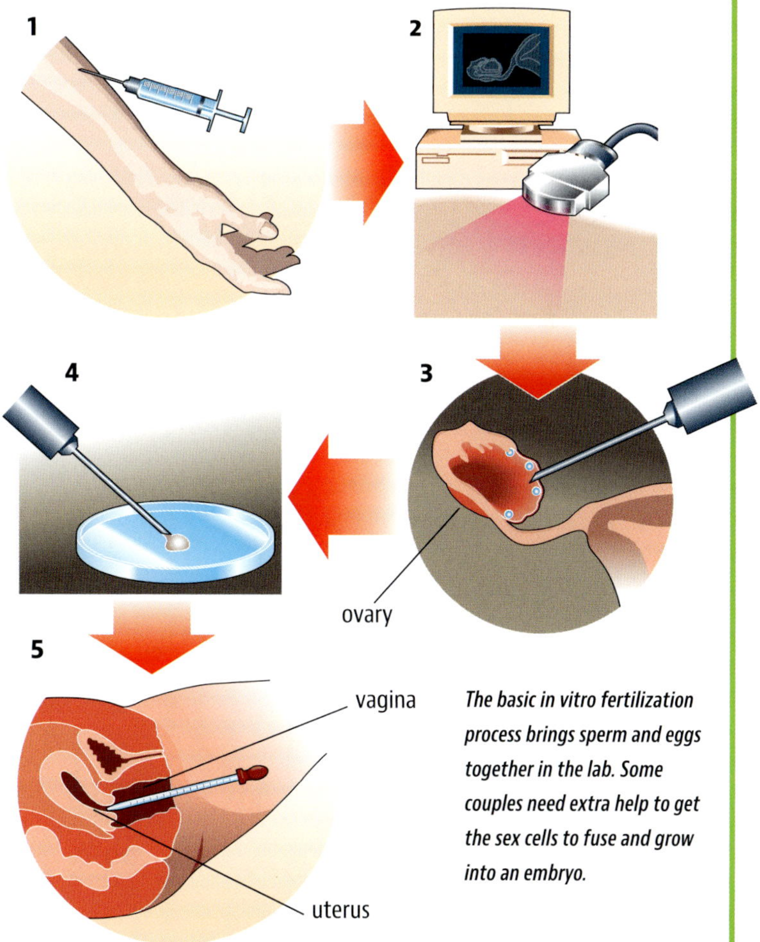

The basic in vitro fertilization process brings sperm and eggs together in the lab. Some couples need extra help to get the sex cells to fuse and grow into an embryo.

GENE THERAPY

Gene therapy is a technique that can repair or replace faulty genes. The first person to be treated was a four-year-old girl called Ashanti DeSilva. She had a genetic disorder called severe combined immunodeficiency (SCID), which meant her immune system did not work properly. Doctors placed copies of a normal gene in her white blood cells to compensate for a faulty gene. Gene therapy is being tested for a number of conditions. It can be used to treat inherited disorders, such as hemophilia, and diseases, such as leukemia.

Gene editing is a procedure that allows scientists to change an organism's DNA. Genetic material can be added, changed, or removed from a particular site. In this way, researchers can change the genetic code.

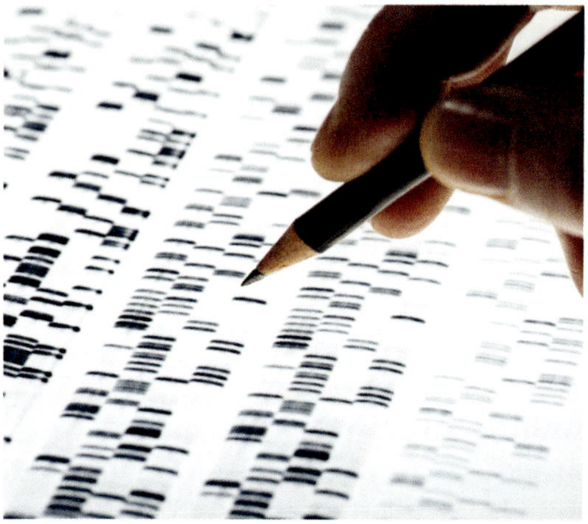

A genetic "fingerprint" is a quick way of revealing genetic makeup. It can be used to confirm relationships between people and to show if a person carries a damaging gene.

CLONING

In 1996 a sheep called Dolly was born in Edinburgh, Scotland. She was the first clone—an identical genetic copy—of an adult mammal.

1 Cells were taken from the udder of an adult ewe. All the body cells of an animal have the same set of genes. However, as the animal develops some unused genes are switched off.
2 A sheep egg cell had its nucleus removed.
3 An electric current fused a nucleus from one of the udder cells with the egg cell, switching all the genes on.
4 The cell became an embryo, which was placed back into a ewe and grew into Dolly—a clone of the ewe from which the udder cells were taken.

It took 277 attempts to make Dolly. She died in 2003 at a much younger age than most sheep. It is unclear whether this was because she was a clone.

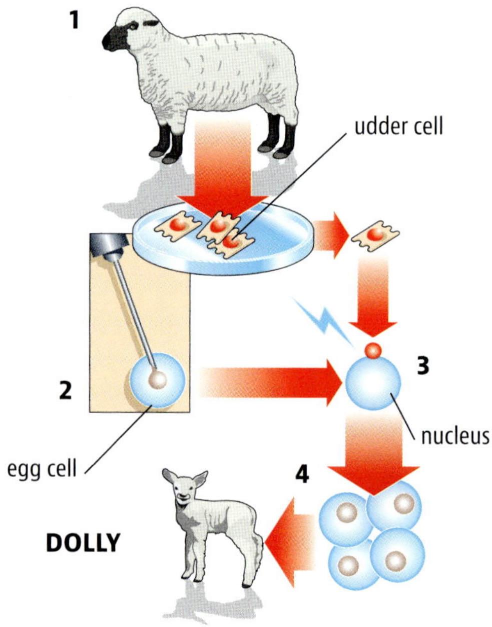

FACTS AND FIGURES

- A person's DNA contains about 20,500 genes. Less than two percent of the DNA carries a code for proteins. The rest is junk, or noncoding, marker units between genes. Scientists still do not understand the role of junk DNA.
- There are two strands of DNA that run in opposite directions to each other.
- The human genome has three million base pairs of DNA arranged into 46 chromosomes.

Identical twins like these have identical sets of genes, which makes them useful subjects in studies into the genetic causes of illnesses. If both twins develop the same disease, then it is likely to have been influenced by their genes.

(the entire genetic code) by locating the position of each gene on particular chromosomes. The project involved hundreds of researchers working to produce a library of all human genes. It was completed in 2003.

Studying the position and chemical nature of a human gene—and any differences between normal and abnormal versions—can help to predict whether a person might become vulnerable to particular diseases, such as heart disease or cancer, in the future. However, many people are worried about the use of such information. If employers or insurance companies demanded genetic screenings, some people might find it harder to get a job or insurance cover if they are found to have an abnormal gene.

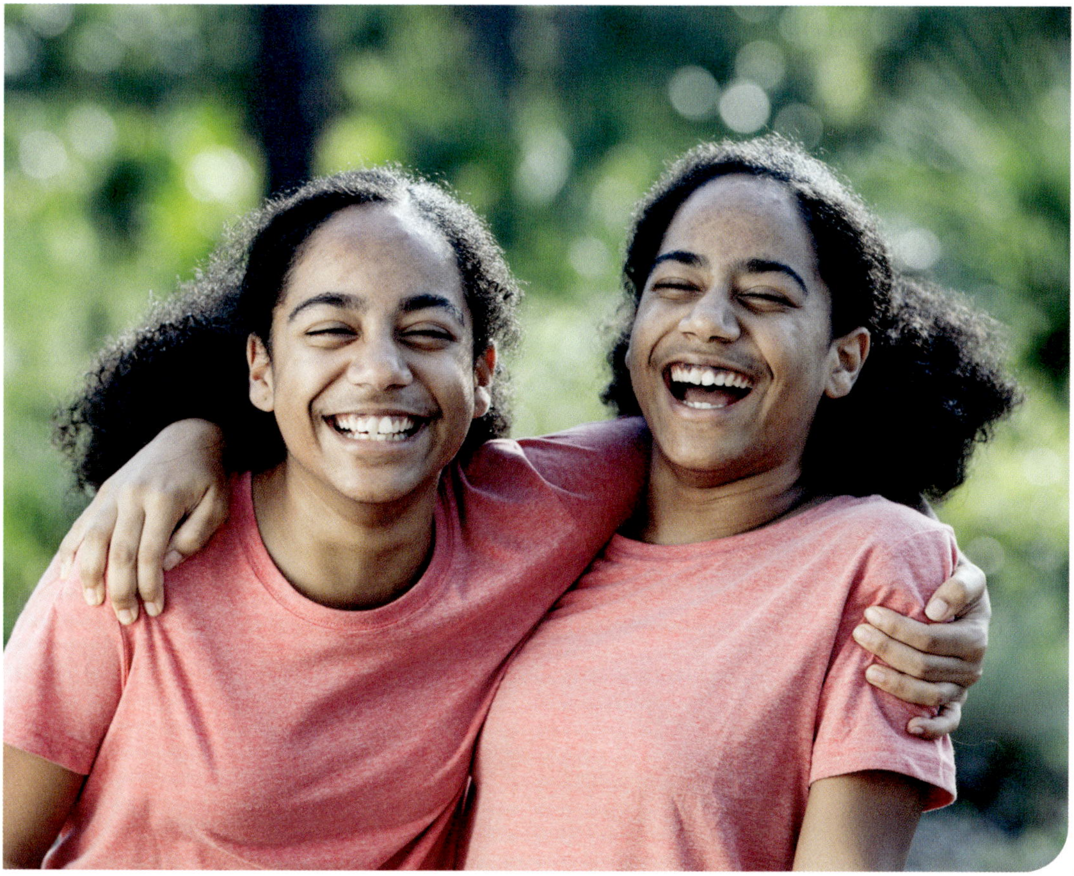

TIMELINE

430 BCE Greek physician Hippocrates develops a new medical technique called clinical observation.

300s BCE Greek doctor Diocles promotes the used of peppermint powder for cleaning teeth.

1543 CE Andreas Vesalius makes many advances in the study of anatomy and publishes his findings in his book, *On the Fabric of the Human Body.*

1592 Galileo Galilei makes the first thermometer.

1600s For almost 30 years, Santorio, an Italian doctor, weighs himself and his food before every meal, and then does the same with his feces, to show that part of the food is extracted by the digestive system.

1628 Physician and anatomist William Harvey discovers the true nature of the circulation of blood inside the body.

1660 Robert Hooke builds a compound microscope and discovers body cells.

1714 Daniel Gabriel Fahrenheit devises the Fahrenheit temperature scale, with the zero measure based on the freezing point of sea water, and the 100 degree mark set at the human body temperature. More accurate measurements showed that a normal body temperature was 98°F (37°C).

1743 Astronomer Anders Celsius invents the Celsius temperature scale with the 0° and 100° points set at the melting and boiling points of pure water.

1795 French chef Nicolas Appert develops a new system of preserving food by heating it in sealed containers.

1816 René Laënnec makes the first stethoscope.

1831 Scientists in the United States, Germany, and France discover the anesthetic properties of chloroform.

1842 Surgeon Crawford Long carries out the first pain-free operation using ether as an anesthetic.

1850s–1880s Microbiologists Louis Pasteur and Robert Koch discover that microorganisms cause many diseases.

1856 Louis Pasteur develops his system of pasteurization.

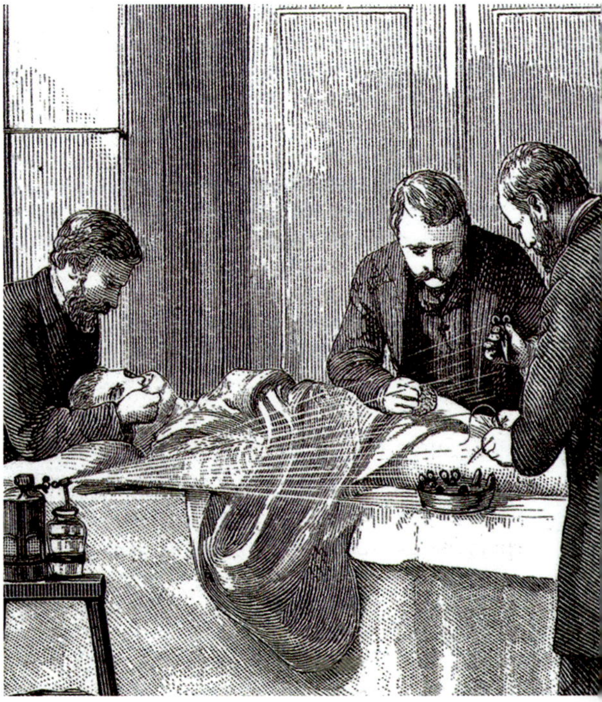

1860s Gregor Mendel studies plant breeding and lays the foundations of genetics.

1865 Joseph Lister performs the first antiseptic operation.

1881 Louis Pasteur demonstrates a vaccine against anthrax.

1910 Salvarsan, the first synthetic chemical drug—discovered by Paul Ehrlich and Sahachiro Hata—goes on commercial sale.

1914 A team at Johns Hopkins Hospital in Baltimore makes the first kidney dialysis machine. Named "the artificial kidney," it was used mainly on dogs.

1928 Alexander Fleming discovers penicillin, an antibiotic. The drug becomes widely used in the 1940s.

1930 John H. Gibbon invents a heart-lung machine.

1952 Physician Robert Lee Wild produces ultrasound images from inside the body.

1953 The structure of deoxyribonucleic acid (DNA) is determined by James Watson and Francis Crick.

1958 The first heart pacemaker is made.

1967 Surgeon Christiaan Barnard carries out the first human-to-human heart transplant.

1972 Janet Mertz and Ron Davis use cut-and-paste techniques to make the first recombinant DNA engineered by humans.

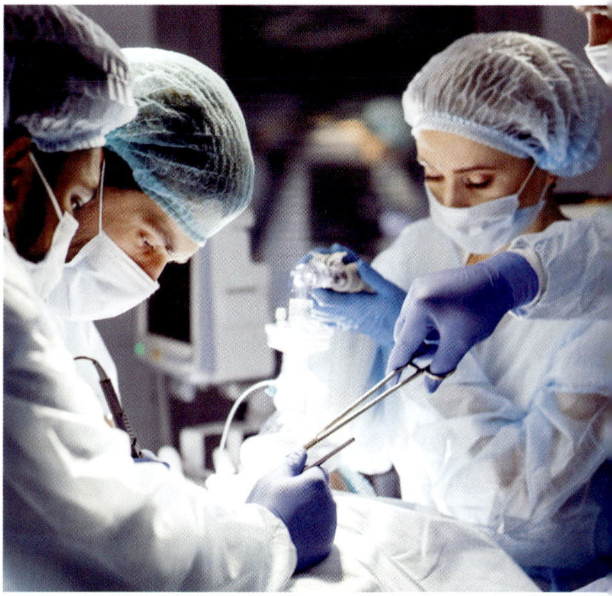

1977 Raymond Damadian takes the first pictures inside the human body using magnetic resonance imaging (MRI).

1996 Dolly the sheep is the first mammal to be successfully cloned.

2003 The Human Genome Project produces an almost complete library of the chemical sequence of every human gene.

2019 China announces it will make researchers and doctors who edit a person's genes personally responsible for any ill effects caused by the treatment.

2020 Emmanuelle Charpentier and Jennifer Doudna are awarded the Nobel Prize for Chemistry for the development of a method for genome editing.

2023 The male contraceptive Pill enters clinical trials.

GLOSSARY

anatomy The arrangement of body parts, such as tissues and organs, inside the body of a living organism, and the science of identifying and describing these parts.

anesthetic A chemical that renders a patient unable to feel pain.

antibody A protein produced by the body's immune system in response to foreign substances, or antigens. Many different types of antibodies are made, each able to bind to a particular antigen. Once antibodies have bound, the antigen can be engulfed and destroyed by white blood cells.

antigen A protein, toxin, or other large molecule to which the body reacts by producing antibodies.

bacteria Single-celled microorganisms that are present almost everywhere on Earth. Bacteria can only be seen through a microscope, and most are spherical, rodlike, or spiral in shape. Some bacteria are beneficial to people, helping us digest our food and playing an important part in the preparation of some foods. Others, however, are responsible for serious diseases such as cholera.

cancer A disease caused when cells divide uncontrollably, forming a tumor.

clone An organism that is genetically identical to its parents and siblings.

chromosome A structure, found inside the nucleus of a cell, that contains DNA.

DNA Deoxyribonucleic acid, a double-stranded molecule that carries genetic information.

electromagnetic radiation Waves made up of electric and magnetic fields. Electromagnetic waves travel at the speed of light, but the characteristics of a particular wave are determined by its frequency. Radio waves and microwaves are low-frequency electromagnetic waves, while infrared, visible light, ultraviolet, and X rays are produced as the frequency increases.

enzyme A biological catalyst—a protein molecule produced by an organism to control or perform a particular chemical reaction.

epidemic A disease outbreak in which people fall ill more quickly than usual.

fermentation The breakdown of sugars to release energy. In certain conditions some types of yeast and other microorganisms release carbon dioxide and alcohol as waste products from fermentation, an effect that is used in breadmaking and brewing.

gene therapy Treatment of a genetic disorder by replacing a faulty gene with a healthy copy.

genetic Relating to, or the study of, the inherited features of an organism.

genome The entire set of genetic information in an organism. It is held in the chromosomes and provides all the information the organism needs to function.

hormone A substance released by certain glands into the bloodstream that travels to and acts on remote sites in the body. Both natural hormones and artificial hormones are often used in medicine.

immunize To protect from the effects of a harmful substance or disease. There are two forms of immunization—passive, which involves injecting the patient with antibodies, and active, in which a form of harmful substance that has been made harmless in some way is injected, allowing the patient to generate antibodies toward it.

Industrial Revolution A great change in social and economic organization brought about by the replacement of hand tools by machines and power tools, and the development of large-scale industrial production methods. The Industrial Revolution started in England around 1760 and spread to the rest of Europe and the United States.

magnetism All phenomena associated with magnets and magnetic fields. Magnetic fields are regions around magnets in which a force acts on any magnet or electric charge present.

magnets Any material capable of generating a magnetic field.

microorganism An organism too small to be seen with the eye alone. For example, bacteria, viruses, and yeasts.

MRI Magnetic Resonance Imaging, a machine that scans the body using magnetic fields and radio waves.

plague A deadly disease that spreads through a population. The Black Death was a disease called bubonic plague, spread by the fleas of rats.

positrons Positively charged subatomic particles with the same mass as electrons. Positrons are very unstable and rapidly react with any matter to form gamma rays.

protons Basic components of atoms. Protons are located in the nucleus and have a positive electric charge.

radioactivity The disintegration of atomic nuclei accompanied by giving off particles or electromagnetic waves.

recombinant DNA DNA molecules that have been created by artificially pasting together DNA fragments that are often taken from different species.

transplant A surgical procedure in which an organ or other body part is moved from one part of the body to another or from one person (the donor) to another (the recipient).

trepanning A primitive surgical procedure in which a hole is cut in the skull to release pressure.

vaccine A medication, often containing disease-causing microorganisms that have been killed or weakened, which is administered to immunize or increase immunity to a particular illness.

virus A tiny, disease-causing particle that consists of protein combined with genetic material (DNA or RNA—ribonucleic acid). Viruses are only capable of replicating inside living cells, and for this reason many scientists do not consider them to be living organisms; other scientists, however, consider them to be a type of microorganism.

white blood cells Components of the blood responsible for destroying foreign substances and organisms. Different types of white blood cells perform different functions in this process, which is called the immune response. Some generate antibodies, while others engulf and digest foreign particles.

X ray A type of electromagnetic radiation with a wavelength between 0.001 and 10 nm. X rays are able to travel through soft tissues and can be used to study the internal structures of the body.

FURTHER RESEARCH

Books

The Complete Human Body: The Definitive Visual Guide by Dr Alice Roberts. New York: Dorling Kindersley, 2023.

Medicine Through the Ages: From Acupuncture to Antibiotics by Michael Woods and Mary Woods. Minneapolis, MN: Lerner Publishing, 2024.

A Short, Illustrated History of Medicine by John C. Miles. New York: Rosen Publishing, 2025.

Web Sites

Science Museum, London: fighting disease
www.sciencemuseum.org.uk/medicine

National Museum and Health and Medicine
www.medicalmuseum.mil/

History of Surgery
www.rasmussen.edu/degrees/health-sciences/blog/history-of-surgery/

INDEX